Milestones in Drug Therapy
MDT

TNF-alpha Inhibitors

Edited by J.M. Weinberg and R. Buchholz

Birkhäuser Verlag
Basel · Boston · Berlin

Editors
Jeffrey M. Weinberg
Robin Buchholz
Department of Dermatology
St. Luke's-Roosevelt Hospital Center
1090 Amsterdam Avenue, Suite 11D
New York, NY 10025
USA

A CIP catalogue record for this book is available from the Library of Congress, Washington D.C., USA

Bibliographic information published by Die Deutsche Bibliothek
Die Deutsche Bibliothek lists this publication in the Deutsche Nationalbibliografie; detailed bibliographic data is available in the internet at http://dnb.ddb.de

ISBN 3-7643-7248-6 Birkhäuser Verlag, Basel - Boston - Berlin

Part of Springer Science+Business Media
Printed on acid-free paper produced from chlorine-free pulp. TFC ∞
Cover illustration: see p. 16. With the friendly permission of Ting Chang and Seth Stevens.

Printed in Germany
ISBN-10: 3-7643-7248-6
ISBN-13: 978-3-7643-7248-4

e-ISBN-10: 3-7643-7438-1
e-ISBN-13: 978-3-7643-7438-9

9 8 7 6 5 4 3 2 1

www. birkhauser.ch

Contents

List of contributors

Andrew F. Alexis, St. Luke's-Roosevelt Hospital, 1090 Amsterdam Avenue Suite 11B, New York, NY 10025, USA; e-mail: andrew.alexis@columbia.edu
Ting H. Chang, Amgen, One Amgen Center Drive, MS 27-4-A, Thousand Oaks, CA 91320, USA; e-mail: tingc@amgen.com
Jennifer Clay Cather, Baylor University Medical Center, Dallas, TX 75231, USA; e-mail: jennifercather@mac.com
Dirk M. Elston, Department of Dermatology, Geisinger Medical Center, 100 North Academy Ave, Danville, PA 17822-1406, USA; e-mail: Delston@geisinger.edu
Harry D. Fischer, Rheumatology, Beth Israel Medical Center, Phillips Ambulatory Care Center, 10 Union Square East, Room 3d, New York, NY 10003 USA; e-mail: hfischer@bethisraelny.org
Noah Gratch, Joan and Sanford Weill Medical College of Cornell University, New York, NY 10021, USA; e-mail: ngratch@yahoo.com
Jeffrey D. Greenberg, NYU Hospital for Joint Diseases, 301 East 17th Street, Suite 1410, New York, NY 10003, USA; e-mail: jeffrey.greenberg@nyumc.org
Mitsumasa Kishimoto, NYU Hospital for Joint Diseases, 301 East 17th Street, Suite 1410, New York, NY 10003, USA; e-mail: kishimotomitsumasa@yahoo.co.jp
Dahlia T. Lainer, David Geffen School of Medicine, UCLA Medical Center and West Los Angeles VAMC, Los Angeles, CA 90095, USA; e-mail: dlainer@mednet.ucla.edu
Patricia Malerich, Department of Dermatology, Geisinger Medical Center, 100 North Academy Ave, Danville, PA 17822-1406, USA; e-mail: pgmalerich@geisinger.edu
Noah Scheinfeld, Department of Dermatology, St. Luke's-Roosevelt Hospital Center, 1090 Amsterdam Avenue, Suite 11D, New York, NY 10025, USA; e-mail: nss32@columbia.edu
Rahul Shukla, McMaster University and Dermatrials Research, 132 Young Street, Hamilton, ON, L8N 1V6, Canada; e-mail: drvender@dermatrials.com
Seth R. Stevens, Amgen, One Amgen Center Drive, MS 27-1-D, Thousand Oaks, CA 91320, USA; e-mail: sstevens@amgen.com
Mihaela B. Taylor, David Geffen School of Medicine, UCLA Medical Center, Los Angeles, CA 90095, USA; e-mail: mitaylor@mednet.ucla.edu
Ronald B. Vender, McMaster University and Dermatrials Research, 132 Young Street, Hamilton, ON, L8N 1V6, Canada; e-mail: drvender@dermatrials.com

Jeffrey M. Weinberg, Department of Dermatology, St. Luke's-Roosevelt Hospital Center, 1090 Amsterdam Avenue, Suite 11D, New York, NY 10025, USA; e-mail: jmw27@columbia.edu

Melodie Young, Baylor Health Care System, Dallas, TX 75231, USA; e-mail: melodiey@baylorhealth.edu

Preface

Over the last decade, the advent of biologic agents has greatly revolutionized therapeutic medicine in the management of chronic inflammatory diseases, such as rheumatoid arthritis, Crohn's disease, and psoriasis. Elucidation of the complex web of cytokine network and the roles of these cytokines in the pathogenesis of inflammatory disorders provided one of the key catalysts for the advancement of targeted biologic therapy in autoimmune and inflammatory diseases.

TNF-α is known to play a crucial role in the pathogenesis of many chronic inflammatory diseases. Elevated levels of TNF-α have been demonstrated in Crohn's disease, psoriasis, psoriatic arthritis, and rheumatoid arthritis, suggesting a role for TNF-α in their pathogenesis. Although TNF-α plays a critical role in the activation of innate and acquired immune responses, the persistence of the immune response and inappropriate production of TNF-α can produce pathological changes resulting from chronic inflammation and tissue damage.

The purpose of this volume is to provide a comprehensive overview of the development, pharmacology, efficacy, and safety of the currently available TNF-α inhibitors – etanercept, infliximab, and adalimumab.

The initial three chapters of the volume provide a background on the field on TNF-α and its inhibition. Chapter 1 provides an introduction to TNF and reviews the pathophysiology of this cytokine. Chapter 2 then presents the history of the development of TNF inhibitors. The pharmacology of these agents is reviewed in Chapter 3.

The next segment of the volume provides an in-depth evaluation of the applications and efficacy of each of the individual TNF-inhibitors. Chapter 4 reviews the use of etanercept in rheumatology, while Chapter 5 surveys the use of this drug in dermatology and off-label applications. Chapter 6 evaluates the use of infliximab in rheumatology, and Chapter 7 reviews its use in dermatology, gastroenterology, and as an off-label agent. Finally, Chapters 8 and 9 discuss the use of adalimumab, respectively, in rheumatology and dermatology.

The final chapter of the book reviews the safety of all three agents, as the TNF inhibitors share a common set of safety concerns. These drugs have proven very safe, compared with traditional agents, but proper knowledge of their safety issues is necessary for their optimal usage.

The use of biologic agents is truly an evolving field. In this volume, an outstanding group of authors have provided the most recent clinical data, encompassing proper applications, efficacy, and safety. We hope that you will find the information useful in the scope of your research or practice. We urge you, however, to keep abreast of this field after reading this volume, as the flow of new information is constant.

Jeffrey M. Weinberg
Robin Buchholz

New York, January 2006

TNF-alpha Inhibitors
Edited by Jeffrey M. Weinberg and Robin Buchholz

Introduction to TNF/pathophysiology of TNF

Patricia Malerich and Dirk M. Elston

Department of Dermatology, Geisinger Medical Center, Danville, PA, USA

Introduction to basic cell to cell communication and cytokines

The complex organization of cellular functions in the human body requires a precise interplay of activity. Cell to cell communications must be sent and received in an efficient system. When the distance over which a signal must travel is greater then an intracellular space, soluble polypeptide factors called cytokines are employed as messenger proteins [1]. Cytokines are small proteins released by cells that trigger specific effects on target cells equipped to respond. Cytokines can be broadly categorized as primary and secondary cytokines. Primary cytokines, such as IL-1 and Tumor Necrosis Factor alpha (TNF-α), are considered part of the innate immune system and can independently initiate inflammatory cascades in human tissues. Secondary cytokines are produced later in the cascade, after the primary cytokines. They have a more limited range of activity.

TNF-α local and systemic effects

TNF-α is an example of a primary cytokine and the model for a family of proteins classified by the diverse biologic activities they produce as well as the similarity of their receptor molecules. TNF-α is a multidimensional cytokine with effects on cellular metabolism, antiviral activities, coagulation processes, growth regulation of cells and insulin response. In this text, we will focus on the broad range of TNF-α effects on inflammation and immunity.

TNF-α was named based on the observed ability to stimulate necrosis of malignant tumors, but was soon found to be an important mediator of cutaneous inflammation. T cells that recognize peptides bound to major histocompatibility complex (MHC) class II molecules have two types: inflammatory CD4 T cells (Th1) and helper CD4 T cells (Th2). Most antimicrobial responses are Th1 responses, involving a characteristic array of cytokines including TNF-α, IL-12, IL-2, IL-6, IL-8, and IFN-gamma. In contrast, Th2 responses are involved in atopy and allergic reactivity as well as the response to some parasites. Typical Th2 cytokines include IL-4, IL-5, IL-9, and IL-13.

Although the evolutionary advantage of a Th1 inflammatory response may be resistance to infections, TNF-α expression is induced in the course of most inflammatory responses in the skin, and many of these inflammatory responses produce pain, itch and suffering. Control of Th1 responses through modification of cytokine activity has dramatically altered the approach to the treatment of a wide range of inflammatory skin disorders. The recognition of psoriasis as a TNF-α-mediated inflammatory disease was pivotal in the development of biological agents for the treatment of psoriasis. TNF-α also plays a pivotal role in psoriatic arthritis, Crohn's disease, and a range of cutaneous inflammatory disorders [2].

Psoriasis is a hyperproliferative disorder, with the proliferation being driven by a complex cascade of inflammatory mediators. Effective therapeutic agents appear to influence the disease primarily by their effects on the inflammatory cascade. Although the interplay of cytokines is complex, the main signal for development of a Th1 response may be interleukin 12 [3, 4]. Some agents used to treat psoriasis have been shown to affect IL-12, and antibodies specifically targeting this cytokine appear promising as antipsoriatic drugs [5]. Most of the effective biological agents that are currently available target TNF-α, and these agents have proved highly effective in managing severe psoriasis.

A shift in the balance from a predominantly Th1 response to a predominantly Th2 response is associated with improvement in psoriasis [6]. Reduced expression of anti-inflammatory cytokines such as IL-1RA and IL-10 has been found in psoriatic plaques, but the antipsoriatic effect of IL-10 may be related to effects on peripheral blood leukocytes rather than a direct effect on keratinocytes [7–9]. Polymorphisms of IL-19 and 20 genes may play a role in the pathogenesis of psoriasis [10]. Polymorphisms for the IL-10 gene predispose towards psoriasis, and a response to therapy is correlated with rising levels of IL-10 mRNA expression [11].

Available biologic agents target CD2-positive lymphocytes, CD-11a and TNF-α, and specific targets for therapy include TNF-α, LFA-1/ICAM-1 binding, and LFA-3/CD2 binding. New agents may target other cytokines, including IL-12 and IL-15. IL-15 promotes recruitment of inflammatory cells in psoriasis, as well as angiogenesis, and the production of additional cytokines [12]. An IL-15 monoclonal antibody appears promising in a mouse model of psoriasis [13]. As most of the currently available agents target TNF-α, a thorough understanding of its function and interactions is critical. This will be the major focus of this chapter.

Interaction of TNF-α with other cytokines

TNF-α induction of cytokine cascades can begin and maintain inflammation. This is evidenced by stimulated release of interleukin-1, interleukin-2, interleukin-6, interleukin-8, granulocyte-macrophage colony-stimulating factor, transforming growth factor and interferon-γ [14–16]. TNF-α may also be involved in apoptosis of aging lymphocytes [17]. An understanding of the complex relationship of cytokines is critical to the development of agents to modify their effects on inflammation and cellular proliferation.

Endothelial cells

TNF-α initiates inflammation by changes in the local vasculature. Endothelial cells treated with TNF-α demonstrate increased production of vasodilators such as prostaglandin and nitric oxide. The resulting increase in tissue perfusion serves to increase the concentration of inflammatory cells in the area. TNF-α amplifies endothelial cell surface L – selectins, E-selectins and P-selectins, and ICAM-1, in turn encouraging tethering, rolling and adhesion of arriving leukocytes [18, 19]. Endothelial cells also begin to secrete cytokines that assist in activation of leukocytes as well as furthering their migration. TNF-α induces vascular endothelial growth factor aiding in vascular permeability, leukocyte migration and creating new vessel networks but the interplay of these factors is complex [20]. The extravasation of activated leukocytes is an active and multifaceted process that coincides with the non-specific movement of fluid out of the vessel through the altered vessel wall. Vascular leakage helps to form a matrix that can be used by leukocytes for extended migration, while induction of matrix metalloproteinases results in destruction of the extracellular matrix. These leukocyte behaviors are intimately associated with the inflammatory response in psoriasis and represent targets for therapy.

Neutrophils

TNF-α enhances accumulation of neutrophils through stimulation of expression of IL-8. Neutrophils may be the major source of IL-8 within psoriatic skin lesions, with autocrine secretion resulting in microabscess and pustule formation [21].

Macrophages

TNF-α is major activator of macrophages, increasing nitric oxide production, proinflammatory cytokines and chemokine production. TNF-α upregulates macrophage inflammatory protein-3 alpha (CCL20) and it's receptor in psoriasis [22]. It also acts to upregulate expression of vascular endothelial growth factor and heme oxygenase-1 [20].

Keratinocytes

TNF-α regulates not only inflammatory responses but also cell motility, cell cycle activity, and apoptosis. The result is increased proliferation of keratinocytes. Interactions with keratinocytes involve an array of chemokines induced by TNF-α. The sum includes promotion of proliferation, and tissue repair by inducing basement membrane components and collagen-degrading proteases. TNF-α induces actin cytoskeleton regulators and integrins, resulting in enhanced keratinocyte motility and attachment [23].

Joint and bone changes

TNF-α stimulates bone and proteoglycan resorption through actions of inflammatory molecules such as prostaglandins and leukotrienes. Cartilage synthesis is not only inhibited but formed cartilage is destroyed by collagenase proteins. TNF-α stimulates neutrophils and fibroblasts to produce a variety of enzymes including collagenase and matrix metalloproteinase that have direct roles in tissue and joint damage [24, 25].

Systemic effects

All the members of the class of cytokines represented by TNF-α are capable of initiating a systemic acute phase reaction. TNF-α treated hepatocytes display an increase in acute phase proteins resulting in systemic effects, such as fever and shock. TNF-α can create tissue and vascular injury by increasing pro-coagulant proteins such as tissue factor and at the same time decreasing anticoagulant proteins. Therefore, TNF-α has been thought to play a prominent role in systemic diseases in which the major component is chronic inflammation, including graft *versus* host disease, bacterial septic shock, and AIDS proliferation of Kaposi's sarcoma cells [26, 27].

TNF and the basic molecular makeup

The TNF-α protein belongs to a trimeric domain protein family, which consists of 18 genes mapped to chromosome position 7p21 that encodes 20 proteins [28]. TNF-α exists in a membrane bound nonglycosylated form and in a soluble form. The soluble and membrane bound forms of TNF-α are both biologically dynamic, differentiated by their affinities for receptors. TNF-α-converting enzyme (TACE) or TNF-α-converting activity (TACA) produces TNF-α by cleaving a 233-amino acid precursor protein and also creates the soluble 17-kDa TNF-α by cleaving the 26-kDa transmembrane TNF-α [29]. As the TNF-α monomers are shed from the cell membrane, they combine into trimolecular complexes (51-kDa homotrimers), consisting of three 17-KDa subunits. These trimers are composed of antiparallel beta pleated sheets folded into a 'jelly roll' structural motif that are then able to bind to the receptors.

Cells that produce TNF

TNF-α is released by a variety of cells including activated keratinocytes, dermal dendrocytes, monocytes and macrophages, mast cells, and activated B and T cells. Activated macrophages comprise the major cellular source of TNF-α. During late phase inflammation, mast cells are capable of increasing TNF-α secretion when induced by Substance P. Keratinocytes in non-inflamed skin can produce TNF-α after exposure to ultraviolet light or bacterial antigens.

Receptor–ligand interaction

There are two receptors for TNF-α: the p55 (CD 120a, tumor necrosis factor receptor -TNFR I, TNF receptor super family member 1A) and p75 receptors (CD 120b, TNFRII, TNF receptor super family member 1B) [29]. Both receptor types can be found on the surface of macrophages, lymphocytes, keratinocytes, and endothelial cells in the blood, as well as the synovial membrane and fluid. The p55 receptor variant is expressed more commonly on cells that are susceptible to the apoptotic destruction, while the p75 receptor variant is increased on activated B cells and T cells. The receptors have the basic membrane structure of an extracellular binding site for TNF-α, a transmembrane domain, and a cytoplasmic tail. There are soluble receptors for TNF-α, possibly shed from mononuclear cells that on a low level appear to act as competitive inhibitors for TNF-α binding to cell surface receptors. All levels of TNF-α receptors are increased following exposure to TNF-α, creating potential for a self-perpetuating positive feedback loop.

The main cellular signaling accomplished by TNF-α is through activation of nuclear transcription factors nuclear factor (NF-κB). NF-κB exists as a heterodimer protein consisting of a 50-kDa (p50) and a 65-kDa (p65) protein subunit [30]. NF-κB resides in the cytosol of inactive cells bound to inhibitor proteins called I kappa B (IκB). In order to create an active signal the inhibitor proteins must be shed from NF-κB by a complex intracellular process of phosphorylation, ubiquitization and proteolytic destruction. The cell membrane binding of the TNF-α cytokine results in an aggregation or multimerization of the receptors to match the trimeric structure of the TNF-α ligand. The ligand–receptor interaction activates an IκB kinase (IKK) complex consisting of two kinase subunits. The IKK complex phosphorylates the IκB inhibitor proteins at the serine residues (S32 and S36) [31]. This creates a target for ubliquitination by E3 ubiquitin ligase complex that marks the IκB inhibitor proteins for proteolytic degradation. Once the inhibitor proteins are destroyed by this process, free NF-κB moves into the nucleus and activates gene transcription through binding to the DNA. NF-κB is a critical regulator of a number of genes which are involved in the inflammation response, including genes producing cytokines, encoding receptors, cell adhesion molecules, growth factors and receptors, and acute-phase proteins.

TNF alpha *versus* TNF beta

Tumor Necrosis Factor (TNF) exists in two forms: TNF-α and TNF-β, also known as lymphotoxin-alpha. These two cytokines have similar functions, but independent cellular origins. TNF-α is secreted by and targets tumor cells and inflammatory cells and induces cytokine induction effects. It is associated with chronic systemic inflammatory response and has also been associated with severe weight loss. T helpers and T cytotoxic cells secrete TNF-β, which creates cytotoxic effects on tumor cells and increase phagocytic activity in macrophages and neutrophil. TNF-β, when compared to TNF-α, is a larger molecule, less plentiful, less effective, produced primarily by T cells and function mostly by direct cytotoxicity to cells [29].

TNF role in psoriasis and psoriatic arthritis

As stated above, psoriasis is an immunologically mediated, hyperproliferative disorder. T cells and cytokines play central roles in the pathophysiology of psoriasis with TNF-α as an essential primary cytokine for cellular signaling during the immune responses. Continued unregulated production of TNF-α as seen in the chronic inflammation of psoriasis and psoriatic arthritis can lead to the consequences of tissue disruption, joint injury, and excessive keratinocyte proliferation by the mechanisms stated above [32]. By self-perpetuated upregulation of receptors, TNF-α creates a positive feedback loop, amplifying and maintaining the inflammatory process within psoriatic plaques. TNF-α induces chemokines that find increased receptors on inflammatory lymphocytes in psoriasis. High levels of TNF-α in psoriatic lesions and in psoriatic arthritis synovial fluid, as well as evidence of correlation of disease severity and TNF-α levels have all provided credibility for the role of TNF-α in psoriasis [33]. Therefore, TNF-α has become a target for therapy in the biologic treatment of psoriasis.

References

1 Chanson M, Derouette JP, Roth I, Foglia B, Scerri I, Dudez T, Kwak BR (2005) Gap junctional communication in tissue inflammation and repair. *Biochim Biophys Acta* 1711(2): 197–207
2 Numerof RP, Dinarello CA, Asadullah K (2005) Cytokines as potential therapeutic targets for

inflammatory skin diseases. *Eur Cytokine Netw* 16(2): 101–103
3 Rodriguez-Galan MC, Bream JH, Farr A, Young HA (2005) Synergistic effect of IL-2, IL-12, and IL-18 on thymocyte apoptosis and Th1/Th2 cytokine expression. *J Immunol* 174(5): 2796–2804
4 Takatori H, Nakajima H, Kagami S, Hirose K, Suto A, Suzuki K, Kubo M, Yoshimura A, Saito Y, Iwamoto I (2005) Stat5a inhibits IL-12-induced Th1 cell differentiation through the induction of suppressor of cytokine signaling 3 expression. *J Immunol* 174(7): 4105–4112
5 Rosmarin D, Strober BE (2005) The potential of interleukin 12 inhibition in the treatment of psoriasis. *J Drugs Dermatol* 4(3): 318–325
6 Ghoreschi K, Rocken M (2004) Immune deviation strategies in the therapy of psoriasis. *Curr Drug Targets Inflamm Allergy* 3(2): 193–198
7 Hammerberg C, Arend WP, Fisher GJ, Chan LS, Berger AE, Haskill JS, Voorhees JJ, Cooper KD (1992) Interleukin-1 receptor antagonist in normal and psoriatic epidermis. *J Clin Invest* 90(2): 571–583
8 Tarlow JK, Cork MJ, Clay FE, Schmitt-Egenolf M, Crane AM, Stierle C, Boehncke WH, Eiermann TH, Blakemore AI, Bleehen SS et al (1997) Association between interleukin-1 receptor antagonist (IL-1ra) gene polymorphism and early and late-onset psoriasis. *Br J Dermatol* 136(1): 147–148
9 Seifert M, Sterry W, Effenberger E, Rexin A, Friedrich M, Haeussler-Quade A, Volk HD, Asadullah K (2000) The antipsoriatic activity of IL-10 is rather caused by effects on peripheral blood cells than by a direct effect on human keratinocytes. *Arch Dermatol Res* 292(4): 164–172
10 Koks S, Kingo K, Ratsep R, Karelson M, Silm H, Vasar E (2004) Combined haplotype analysis of the interleukin-19 and -20 genes: relationship to plaque-type psoriasis. *Genes Immun* 5(8): 662–667
11 Kingo K, Koks S, Silm H, Vasar E (2003) IL-10 promoter polymorphisms influence disease severity and course in psoriasis. *Genes Immun* 4(6): 455–457
12 McInnes IB, Gracie JA (2004) Interleukin-15: a new cytokine target for the treatment of inflammatory diseases. *Curr Opin Pharmacol* 4(4): 392–397
13 Villadsen LS, Schuurman J, Beurskens F, Dam TN, Dagnaes-Hansen F, Skov L, Rygaard J, Voorhorst-Ogink MM, Gerritsen AF, van Dijk MA et al (2003) Resolution of psoriasis upon blockade of IL-15 biological activity in a xenograft mouse model. *J Clin Invest* 112(10): 1571–1580
14 Saripalli YV, Gaspari AA (2005) Focus on: biologics that affect therapeutic agents in dermatology. *J Drugs Dermatol* 4(2): 233–245
15 Goldsmith DR, Wagstaff AJ (2005) Etanercept: a review of its use in the management of plaque psoriasis and psoriatic arthritis. *Am J Clin Dermatol* 6(2): 121–136
16 Singh R, Robinson DB, El-Gabalawy HS (2005) Emerging biologic therapies in rheumatoid arthritis: cell targets and cytokines. *Curr Opin Rheumatol* 17(3): 274–279
17 Gupta S, Gollapudi S (2005) Molecular mechanisms of TNF-alpha-induced apoptosis in aging human T cell subsets. *Int J Biochem Cell Biol* 37(5): 1034–1042
18 Keystone E (2004) Adalimumab therapy in rheumatoid arthritis. *Rheum Dis Clin North Am* 30(2): 349–364, vii
19 Yang L, Froio RM, Sciuto TE, Dvorak AM, Alon R, Luscinskas FW (2005) ICAM-1 regulates neutrophil adhesion and transcellular migration of TNF-{alpha} activated vascular endothelium under flow. *Blood* 5 106: 584–589
20 Malaguarnera L, Imbesi R, Di Rosa M, Scuto A, Castrogiovanni P, Messina A, Sanfilippo S (2005) Action of prolactin, IFN-gamma, TNF-alpha and LPS on heme oxygenase-1 expression and VEGF release in human monocytes/macrophages. *Int Immunopharmacol* 5(9): 1458–1469
21 Duan H, Koga T, Kohda F, Hara H, Urabe K, Furue M (2001) Interleukin-8-positive neutrophils in psoriasis. *J Dermatol Sci* 26(2): 119–124
22 Homey B, Dieu-Nosjean MC, Wiesenborn A, Massacrier C, Pin JJ, Oldham E, Catron D, Buchanan ME, Muller A, deWaal Malefyt R et al (2000) Up-regulation of macrophage inflammatory protein-3 alpha/CCL20 and CC chemokine receptor 6 in psoriasis. *J Immunol* 164(12): 6621–6632
23 Banno T, Gazel A, Blumenberg M (2004) Effects of tumor necrosis factor-alpha (TNF alpha) in epidermal keratinocytes revealed using global transcriptional profiling. *J Biol Chem* 279(31): 32633–32642
24 Myers W, Opeola M, Gottlieb AB (2004) Common clinical features and disease mechanisms of psoriasis and psoriatic arthritis. *Curr Rheumatol Rep* 6(4): 306–313
25 Anandarajah AP, Ritchlin CT (2004) Pathogenesis of psoriatic arthritis. *Curr Opin Rheumatol*

16(4): 338–343
26 Pryhuber GS, Huyck HL, Roper JM, Cornejo J, O'Reilly MA, Pierce RH, Tsitsikov EN (2005) Acute tumor necrosis factor-{alpha}-induced liver injury in the absence of tumor necrosis factor receptor-associated factor 1 gene expression. *Am J Pathol* 166(6): 1637–1645
27 Carlson DL, Willis MS, White DJ, Horton JW, Giroir BP (2005) Tumor necrosis factor-alpha-induced caspase activation mediates endotoxin-related cardiac dysfunction. *Crit Care Med* 33(5): 1021–1028
28 Najarian DJ (2003) Connections between psoriasis and Crohn's disease. *J Am Acad Dermatol* 48(6): 805–821
29 Babu KS (2004) Role of tumor necrosis factor alpha in asthma. Immunol Allergy Clin North *Am* 24(4): 583–597, v–vi
30 Beg AA, Finco TS, Nantermet PV, Baldwin AS Jr, (1993) Tumor necrosis factor and interleukin-1 lead to phosphorylation and loss of IκBα: A mechanism for NF-κB activation. *Mol Cell Biol* 13: 3301–3310
31 Loop T (2003) Thiopental inhibits tumor necrosis factor alpha-induced activation of nuclear factor kappaB through suppression of kappaB kinase activity. *Anesthesiology* 99(2): 360–367
32 Gottlieb AB (2003) Pharmacodynamic and pharmacokinetic response to anti-tumor necrosis factor-alpha monoclonal antibody (infliximab) treatment of moderate to severe psoriasis vulgaris. *J Am Acad Dermatol* 48(1): 68–75
33 Yamauchi PS (2004) The treatment of psoriasis and psoriatic arthritis with etanercept: practical considerations on monotherapy, combination therapy, and safety. *Dermatol Clin* 22(4): 449–459, ix

TNF-alpha Inhibitors
Edited by Jeffrey M. Weinberg and Robin Buchholz

History of development of TNF inhibitors

Seth R. Stevens and Ting H. Chang

Amgen, Thousand Oaks, California, USA

Introduction

Over the last decade, the advent of biologic agents has greatly revolutionized therapeutic medicine in the management of chronic inflammatory diseases, such as rheumatoid arthritis (RA), Crohn's disease, and psoriasis. Elucidation of the complex web of cytokine network and the roles of these cytokines in the pathogenesis of inflammatory disorders provided one of the key catalysts for the advancement of targeted biologic therapy in autoimmune diseases.

Cytokines are low molecular weight glycoproteins or small polypeptides that act as intercellular messenger molecules and function in a number of processes, including host defense, tissue growth, repair, and control of neoplasms [1]. Cellular and molecular studies during the 1980s and 1990s have shown strong evidence that immunologic cells (e.g., T lymphocytes, macrophages) and cells that are not typically considered to be immunocytes (e.g., keratinocytes, fibroblasts) produce a wide spectrum of cytokines during the course of an immune response [1]. Because each cytokine has the ability to regulate its own expression as well as the expression of other cytokines in an autocrine and paracrine fashion [1, 2], the inflammatory response is often amplified through a cascade of signaling events, and therefore, must be tightly controlled. One such mechanism is the concomitant production of proinflammatory cytokines (e.g., interleukin 1 [IL-1], interferon γ [INF-γ]) that potentiate the inflammatory response and anti-inflammatory cytokines (e.g., IL-1 receptor antagonists, IL-4), which function to limit the duration and extent of the proinflammatory effect, in essence maintaining a level of homeostasis [2, 3].

While the causes of many chronic inflammatory diseases are unknown, most are characterized by dysregulation of cytokine networks, which often leads to the overproduction of proinflammatory cytokines, thus perturbing the equilibrium between pro- and anti-inflammatory cytokines [2, 4, 5]. At the apex of this cytokine network is tumor necrosis factor-α (TNF-α), which acts as the primary trigger for the inflammatory response by promoting the synthesis of other proinflammatory cytokines [2, 6, 7]. Since its cloning in the mid-1980s, TNF-α has been studied extensively for its biochemical and biological properties [8–10]. These studies have shown that human TNF-α is produced primarily by monocytes/macrophages as a 26 kDa membrane proprotein, which is subsequently cleaved by the TNF-α converting enzyme (TACE) in the extracellular domain to release the mature, 17 kDa, soluble TNF monomer [11, 12]. The active form of TNF-α is a homotrimer that binds to its ubiquitous cognate receptors, TNFRs (p55 and p75). TNFRs can also be cleaved by TACE to produce soluble TNFRs, which function as modulators of TNF activity [2, 13, 14].

TNF-α was originally characterized simultaneously as a factor that produced tumor hemorrhagic necrosis *in vivo* and exhibited anti-tumor activity *in vitro*, through what is now known as programmed cell death or apoptotic pathways [6, 9]. Because of its ability to induce apoptosis in some cancerous or transformed cell lines, TNF-α was considered a potential agent for cancer therapy. However, enthusiasm waned and recognition that anti-tumor properties were minimal when a number of studies in several malignant diseases showed that TNF-α provided no therapeutic benefits for cancer patients, but was instead associated with severe side effects [15, 16]. Since the cloning of TNF-α and a homologous gene, lymphotoxin α (LT-α, also named TNF-β), 19 other TNF ligands and 29 TNFRs have since been identified, including TNF-related apoptosis-inducing ligand (TRAIL) [17–19]. It is now recognized that members of the TNF family have pleiotropic effects on many cellular processes, including programmed cell death (or apoptosis), inflammation, and angiogenesis [17]. That some members, such as TRAIL, are strong inducers of tumor cytotoxicity, but lack toxicity to normal tissues, suggests that these cytokines may be better candidates for cancer therapy than TNF-α.

In hindsight, the name tumor necrosis factor was perhaps a misnomer given that the real role of TNF-α in immunology was less likely immune surveillance of incipient neoplasms, but rather the early and primary orchestration of the inflammatory response. According to this paradigm, it is not surprising then that recombinant TNF-α had proven to be so toxic in clinical trials since administration of the cytokine most likely sent the immune system into overdrive, similar to shock. It soon became apparent to researchers (such as Craig Smith at Immunex) that elevated TNF-α production was a major driver of chronic inflammation characterizing autoimmune diseases, and that inhibition of TNF-α could be therapeutically useful. This idea was further supported by studies in which elevated levels of tissue or plasma TNF-α were found in a variety of infections and inflammatory diseases, as well as in other immune diseases associated with sepsis syndrome and Acquired Immune Deficiency Syndrome (AIDS) [1, 20, 21]. Clinical interests in TNF-α subsequently shifted to inflammatory and autoimmune diseases. In this chapter, we provide a historical perspective on the development of two distinct classes of TNF inhibitors, a fully human, soluble p75 TNF-α receptor (Enbrel® [etanercept]) [22] and two monoclonal antibodies to TNF-α (Remicade® [infliximab] and Humira® [adalimumab]) [23, 24]. The development of TNF inhibitors, however, cannot be viewed in isolation but rather in the larger context of an anti-cytokine therapeutic approach. We present different strategies for anti-cytokine therapies that have evolved as a result of the success of anti-TNF therapy.

Early proof-of-concept studies

Because of its prominent role in the cytokine hierarchy, targeting TNF-α seemed like a logical choice for treating inflammatory diseases. However, TNF-α is only one of several cytokines, including IL-1 and IL-6, which are highly elevated in diseased tissues. In addition, because of cytokine redundancy, there were initial doubts that blocking one cytokine would have any biological effects. How, then, did TNF-α evolve into a therapeutic target that formed the basis for the discovery of TNF inhibitors for the treatment of inflammatory diseases?

One of the first clues that TNF-α might be a good therapeutic target came from observations that 1) TNF-α is the earliest cytokine produced by macrophages during an inflammatory response and 2) TNF-α appears to be the primary inducer of other cytokines, including IL-1 [25]. That IL-1 was also implicated in RA pathogenesis provided a strong indication that TNF-α may be key to understanding the molecular pathology of RA. Indeed, the discovery and cloning of soluble forms of TNFRs was both timely and crucial for exploring the clinical value of TNF inhibition in pathological settings such as RA [26].

Rodent models that mimic human RA provided strong evidence of the promise of TNF inhibitors. Lewis rats immunized with methylated bovine serum albumin (mBSA) in complete Freund's adjuvant developed antigen-induced arthritis when challenged with mBSA in the knee joints [27]. Similarly, collagen-type II-induced arthritis in the genetically susceptible DBA-1 strain of mice shared many histopathologic features of human RA, and had highly elevated levels of TNF-α during the disease course [27]. Exogenous injections of TNF-α exacerbated the disease in these models. In both Lewis rats and collagen-induced arthritic mice, TNF-α blockade using either soluble monomeric or dimeric forms of the TNF-α receptor Fc fusion protein reduced the extent and severity of the arthritis and the cellular infiltrates in the joints, with the dimeric form showing dramatic effects.

The importance of TNFRs in the inflammatory response was subsequently confirmed in transgenic mice. In genetically altered mice overexpressing a modified human TNF-α transgene, spontaneous RA-like lesions developed in the joints that consequently led to progressive inflammation, cellular hyperplasia, and bone erosion [28]. Elevated levels of TNF, IL-1, and IL-6 expression were observed in the synovium. In addition, transgenic mice that expressed only a cell-associated form of TNF-α, which is resistant to TACE processing, also spontaneously developed an RA-like phenotype [29]. When these mice were backcrossed into knockout strains of TNFR p55 or TNFR p75 mice, the severity of the arthritis was reduced, indicating that TNF receptors were important for potentiating disease activity.

The success of soluble TNFR Fc fusion proteins to inhibit the inflammatory response and alleviate the signs and symptoms of arthritis in mice and rat models indicated that inhibition of a single proinflammatory cytokine such as

TNF-α could block the generation of dysregulation of a complex cytokine network and may be a useful therapeutic option in inflammatory diseases. This provided the impetus for the development of anti-TNF therapy in the treatment of human RA and other inflammatory diseases. Soon thereafter, monoclonal antibodies directed against TNF-α were also developed, and were similarly shown in arthritic mouse models to reduce the severity of the arthritis [30–32].

Different approaches to TNF inhibition

A number of studies have shown that inhibition of the TNF pathway can be achieved using different approaches, whether by blocking TNF-α mRNA synthesis (via phosphodiesterase inhibitors, prostanoids, thalidomide, or antisense olionucleotides) [33–36], post-translational processing (via TACE and other metalloproteinase inhibitors) [37], or by blocking TNF-α activation of their receptors (via monoclonal antibodies or soluble receptors; Fig. 1). Among these, the latter strategy has proven to be generally effective and safe in the treatment of moderate to severe RA, juvenile RA, Crohn's disease, ankylosing spondylitis, psoriatic arthritis, and moderate to severe psoriasis.

Although TNF inhibitors share the ability to alter the cytokine cascade responsible for perpetuating inflammation in RA and other inflammatory diseases, soluble receptors differ from monoclonal antibodies in substantial ways, not only in how they are produced, but also with regards to their mechanisms of action. For example, emerging evidence suggests that the anti-TNF antibodies, but not soluble receptors, can form large immune complexes that inter-

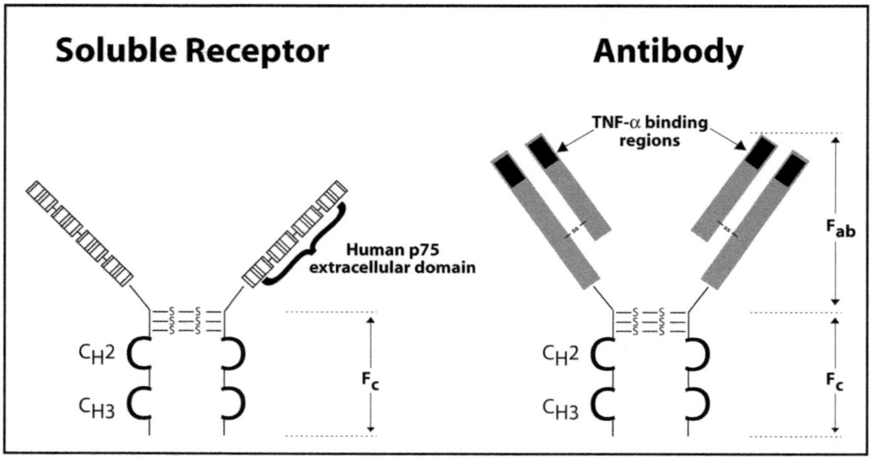

Figure 1. TNF Inhibitors: Soluble TNF receptor and monoclonal antibody. Currently, two classes of TNF inhibitors are approved for use in rheumatoid arthritis, a fully human, soluble TNF receptor (etanercept [Enbrel®]) and two monoclonal antibodies to TNF (infliximab [Remicade®] and adalimumab [Humira®]).

act with C1q and with Fc receptors [38]. Currently, three TNF inhibitors are approved for use in humans: infliximab, adalimumab, and etanercept.

Monoclonal antibodies

Infliximab is a chimeric anti-TNF-α human IgG1κ antibody linked to a variable region of a murine anti-human TNF-α antibody [39]. It was developed based on the success of monoclonal antibodies in arthritic mouse models, and is produced by hybridoma cells. Infliximab binds to both soluble and membrane-bound TNF-α and is able to mediate complement-dependent killing of TNF-expressing cells [40, 41]. However, infusions of infliximab have been shown to induce the development of neutralizing human anti-chimeric antibodies (HACA), which may reduce the clinical efficacy of infliximab therapy [42]. Thus, infliximab must be taken concomitantly with methotrexate, which suppresses HACA development [23].

Adalimumab, another antibody-based therapy, is the most recently introduced TNF inhibitor [24]. It is a fully human IgG anti-TNF-α monoclonal antibody initially developed using phage display and is potentially less immunogenic than infliximab. However, *in vitro*, adalimumab binds to both soluble and membrane-bound TNF-α, and as an antibody, it has the potential to cause cell lysis of surface TNF-expressing cells when complement is present. Like infliximab, adalimumab is also produced by hybridoma cells. Neutralizing antibodies against infliximab and adalimumab have been observed in a subset of patients receiving these anti-TNF-α therapies, which may be associated with reduced efficacy [23, 24].

Soluble receptors

As previously discussed, rodent models have suggested that soluble forms of TNFRs can suppress TNF-α-mediated arthropathy. Etanercept is an engineered dimer of the extracellular portion of the human p75 TNF-α receptor fused to the Fc portion of IgG1, and is produced by Chinese hamster ovary (CHO) mammalian cells [22, 43]. Smith and colleagues identified the gene encoding the p75 receptor by direct expression screening of a human lung fibroblast library [26]. Because the ligand is trimeric, these researchers postulated that the best TNF inhibitor should take a bivalent form – i.e., as a TNFR Fc fusion protein. This crucial design increased both the affinity and serum half-life by orders of magnitude over the monomeric form.

Etanercept binds to both TNF-α and lymphotoxin-α, a related member of the TNF family of cytokines that also activates the inflammatory pathway through the TNFRs [6]. Etanercept does not cause the formation of neutralizing antibodies and does not mediate antibody-dependent cell lysis [22]. The clinical significance of this is unknown. However, while all anti-TNF agents inhibit the TNF pathway, the mechanism of action of each inhibitor may be attributable to significant differences between them. For example, while infliximab is effective in treating Crohn's disease [44], etanercept has not shown therapeutic effects in this indication [45]. Differences in these therapeutic modalities may also account for differences in infection rates between etanercept and the monoclonal antibodies [46]. These differences may also explain why it is possible for patients who have failed therapy with an anti-TNF-α monoclonal antibody to switch to etanercept, and *vice versa*, and still achieve significant clinical response [47, 48].

Another interesting distinction between antibodies and soluble receptors that neutralize cytokines is that while the cytokine-binding portions of soluble receptors are well conserved from individual to individual, and indeed across species, the cytokine-binding portion of monoclonal antibodies are immunologically novel. Thus, while no neutralizing antibodies against etanercept have been detected in treated patients or human subjects, both adalimumab and infliximab engender such antibodies [22–24].

Biologic approaches to cytokine blockade

The success of TNF inhibitors in treating inflammatory disorders led to the development of other anti-cytokine therapies. Unlike immunosuppressants and other traditional therapies that were discovered through serendipity, the development of agents that block cytokine signaling pathways, such as inhibitors of TNF-α, represents a rational treatment approach based on the understanding of the pathophysiology of immune-mediated inflammatory disorders. However, because of the plethora of cytokines that are upregulated during inflammation and in a variety of diseased tissues, identifying which cytokine or cytokine receptor to target posed a great dilemma. Biologic approaches in immune therapy that target cytokine blockade have been largely centered on disease-specific cytokines, as shown in Table 1. Different strategies have been devised, most with the goal of preventing cytokine-receptor signaling activation (Fig. 2). These included the use of soluble receptors, immunoregulatory cytokines, receptor antagonists, and monoclonal antibodies.

Soluble receptors

In theory, soluble receptors with high affinities for specific cytokines can be used to competitively bind and sequester these cytokines away from endogenous receptors (Fig. 2). This approach has been used most successfully in treating TNF-mediated chronic disorders. Studies of TNF-α have demonstrated that under physiological conditions, soluble TNFRs are present in body fluids at ng/mL concentrations and act as inhibitors of TNF-α signaling [13, 14]. Because of the inherent inhibitory nature of soluble TNFRs, it was recognized

Table 1. Anti-cytokine therapies for immune diseases

Anti-cytokine therapy	Therapeutic type	Approved indication
Anti-TNF-α therapy		
Etanercept	Soluble p75 TNF-α receptor	RA, Juvenile RA, psoriasis, AS, PsA
Onercept	Soluble p55 TNF-α receptor	Discontinued (originally developed for psoriasis, PsA, Crohn's disease)
Lenercept	Soluble p55 TNF-α receptor	Discontinued (originally developed for RA and MS)
CDP870	PEGylated anti-TNF antibody	RA
Infliximab	Monoclonal antibody	RA, Crohn's disease, AS, PsA (in development for psoriasis)
Adalimumab	Monoclonal antibody	RA (in development for psoriasis and PsA)
Talidomide of pentoxifylline	Glutamic acid derivative	Leprosy symptoms (in development for RA, lupus, and IBD)
Metalloproteinase inhibitors	Natural or synthetic compounds	In development for RA
TNF-α peptidomimetics	Small molecule peptides	In development for RA
Anti-IL-1 therapy		
Kineret	IL-1 receptor antagonist	RA
Anti-IL-4 therapy		
Pascolizumab	Monoclonal antibody	Discontinued (originally developed for asthma)
Anti-IL-5 therapy		
Mepolizumab	Monoclonal antibody	In development for asthma
Anti-IL-6 therapy		
CNTO-328	Monoclonal antibody	In development for Castleman disease
Anti-IL-10 therapy		
B-N10	Monoclonal antibody	In development for systemic lupus erythematosus
Anti-IL-15 therapy	Monoclonal antibody	In development for RA and psoriasis
Anti-IL-18 therapy	Monoclonal antibody	In development for RA
Recombinant IL-10	Immunoregulatory protein	In development for psoriasis and PsA
Recombinant IL-11	Immunoregulatory protein	In development for psoriasis and PsA
Anti-INF-α therapy		
Antiferon	Monoclonal antibody	In development for AIDS
IFN-β	Immunoregulatory protein	MS

RA = rheumatoid arthritis; AS = ankylosing spondylitis; PsA = psoriatic arthritis; MS = multiple sclerosis; IBD = inflammatory bowel disease

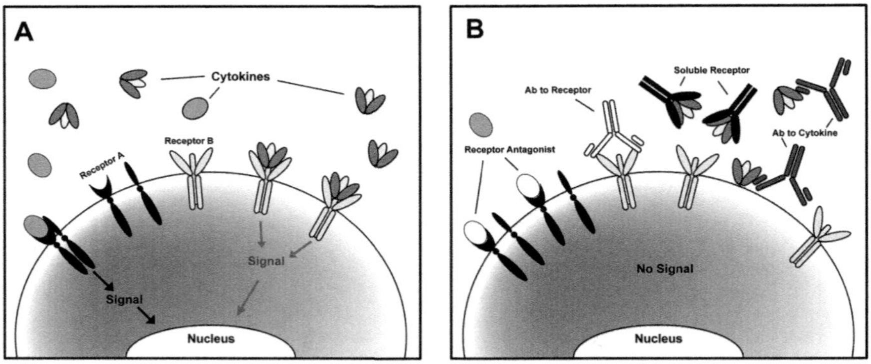

Figure 2. Biologic approaches to cytokine blockade. A) The immune-mediated inflammatory system is comprised of many different cytokines and cytokine receptors, of which two generic pathways are depicted. B) Targeted inhibition of these cytokine pathways can be achieved through various approaches that prevent cytokine-receptor binding, including *receptor antagonists*, *soluble receptors*, and *monoclonal antibodies* to endogenous cytokines or receptors. Abbreviations: Ab = antibody

early on that overproduction of these soluble receptors could be used as a potential form of therapy. Thus, p75 and p55 TNFR Fc fusion proteins, which have high affinities for TNF-α, were developed and tested in humans (Tab. 1). Etanercept was first evaluated in clinical trials in patients with sepsis [49], but did not demonstrate therapeutic benefits. Since then, however, etanercept has been successfully used to treat a number of rheumatic and dermatologic diseases, including moderate to severe RA, juvenile RA, ankylosing spondylitis, moderate to severe psoriasis, and psoriatic arthritis (Tab. 1) [50–54]. Onercept, a p55 receptor, was originally developed for the treatment of psoriasis, psoriatic arthritis, and Crohn's disease [55]; however, recently this program has been halted. Another p55 TNFR, lenercept, was effective in animal models, but did not show clinical efficacy in RA patients [56, 57]. It has been postulated that the lack of efficacy may be due to the immunogenicity of lenercept *in vivo*.

Other soluble receptors, such as the IL-4 receptor (IL-4R) and IL-5R, are currently in development for the treatment of asthma and allergic airway hyper-reactivity, while soluble IFN-γR is being developed for treating patients with autoimmune diabetes [58].

Immunoregulatory cytokines

In inflammatory diseases, overproduction of proinflammatory cytokines can perpetuate the inflammation despite the presence of anti-inflammatory cytokines (e.g., IL-10, IL-11, and IFN-β). Therefore, overproduction of anti-inflammatory cytokines, which negatively regulate the proinflammatory response, may restore the balance between these two classes of cytokines. In clinical trials, administration of IL-11 did not show efficacy compared with placebo in patients with RA [59]. However, treatment with recombinant human IL-10 and IL-11 did improve skin diseases in psoriatic patients [60, 61]. Recombinant IFN-γ has shown efficacy in the treatment of atopic dermatitis, for up to 2 years of continuous therapy [62]. In addition, the use of recombinant IFN-β provided significant reductions in the frequency of multiple sclerosis (MS) attacks, and is now a standard therapy for this indication [63].

Receptor antagonists

Receptor antagonists are naturally occurring molecular species that negatively regulate cytokine signaling activities [6]. One of the most extensively studied receptor antagonist is the IL-1 receptor antagonist (IL-1 Ra), which adheres to IL-1R and blocks the binding of IL-1 [6, 64].

Based on animal studies and studies of RA synoviocytes, IL-1 has been implicated in the pathogenesis and pathology of RA, similar to TNF-α [6, 65, 66]. In fact, IL-1 and TNF-α are thought to share several biologic actions, and can induce the production of one another [6, 65, 66]. While there may be overlapping functions between these two cytokines, IL-1 has shown greater potency than TNF-α in stimulating proteoglycan, a strong inducer of bone and cartilage degradation, when injected in mice [64, 66]. Thus, the balance between IL-1 and IL-1 Ra is important for those with RA.

In the RA joint, overproduction of IL-1 cannot be sufficiently countered by endogenous IL-1 Ra. However, in mouse models, administration of recombinant IL-1 Ra showed strong neutralization of IL-1α and IL-1β, and the inhibition of proteoglycan synthesis [67]. These studies demonstrated that anti-IL-1 therapy was deserving of attention, and led to the development of anakinra (Kineret®), a recombinant, nonglycosylated form of IL-1 Ra, that is approved for use in the treatment of RA [68].

Monoclonal antibodies to cytokines or receptors

By far, monoclonal antibodies have been the most widely used form of anti-cytokine therapy, given their high specificity for their targets. While it seems plausible that monoclonal antibodies should be able to block signaling activities by targeting either the cytokines or their receptors (Fig. 2), to date, most therapies have shown a propensity for targeting the cytokines. As shown in Table 1, monoclonal antibodies directed against IL-4, IL-5, IL-6, IL-10, and IFN-α, are currently at various clinical stages of development for use in a wide-ranging array of inflammatory diseases, including RA, asthma, and systemic lupus erythematosus (SLE) [69–73]. Other promising targets for RA also include IL-15 and IL-18, although these therapies are in early stages of development [74, 75].

Much like soluble TNF-α receptors, monoclonal antibody-based therapies that target TNF-α have also shown clinical efficacy. Infliximab is approved for use in patients with moderate to severe RA, ankylosing spondylitis, psoriatic arthritis, and Crohn's disease [44, 76, 77]. The latest TNF inhibitor approved for use in moderate to severe RA is adalimumab [78]. A PEGylated anti-TNF antibody Fab' fragment, referred to as CDP870, was recently evaluated in a small clinical trial of patients with RA and demonstrated clinical efficacy [79].

Concluding remarks

Advancements in anti-cytokine therapy have been heralded as a new era in the treatment of autoimmune diseases. Insights gained from the development of TNF inhibitors have helped pave the way for the development of other anti-cytokine therapies, which are now in various phases of clinical trials. The success of TNF inhibitors in treating a number of inflammatory illnesses has greatly advanced our understanding of the mechanisms underlying the pathogenesis of these diseases, and raised expectations about the potential for long-term abatement and control of diseases such as moderate to severe RA and psoriasis. Because of these advancements, anti-TNF-α therapies are currently being investigated in patients with other chronic conditions, including congestive heart failure, vasculitis, Behcet's disease, hepatitis, and dermatomyositis.

Acknowledgements
We would like to thank Dr. Craig A. Smith and Dr. Ralph Zitnik, MD, for thoughtful discussions.

References

1 Andreakos ET, Foxwell BM, Brennan FM, Maini RN, Feldmann M (2002) Cytokines and anti-cytokine biologicals in autoimmunity: present and future. *Cytokine Growth Factor Rev* 13: 299–313
2 Feldmann M, Maini RN (2001) Anti-TNF alpha therapy of rheumatoid arthritis: what have we learned? *Annu Rev Immunol* 19: 163–196
3 Arend WP, Dayer JM (1995) Inhibition of the production and effects of interleukin-1 and tumor necrosis factor alpha in rheumatoid arthritis. *Arthritis Rheum* 38: 151–160
4 Asadullah K, Sterry W, Volk HD (2002) Analysis of cytokine expression in dermatology. *Arch Dermatol* 138: 1189–1196
5 Feldmann M, Maini RN (2002) Discovery of TNF-alpha as a therapeutic target in rheumatoid arthritis: preclinical and clinical studies. *Joint Bone Spine* 69: 12–18
6 Borish LC, Steinke JW (2003) 2. Cytokines and chemokines. *J Allergy Clin Immunol* 111: S460–S475
7 van den Berg WB (2001) Anti-cytokine therapy in chronic destructive arthritis. *Arthritis Res* 3: 18–26
8 Aggarwal BB, Aiyer RA, Pennica D, Gray PW, Goeddel DV (1987) Human tumour necrosis factors: structure and receptor interactions. *Ciba Found Symp* 131: 39–51
9 Haranaka K, Carswell EA, Williamson BD, Prendergast JS, Satomi N, Old LJ (1986) Purification, characterization, and antitumor activity of nonrecombinant mouse tumor necrosis factor. *Proc Natl Acad Sci USA* 83: 3949–3953
10 Pennica D, Hayflick JS, Bringman TS, Palladino MA, Goeddel DV (1985) Cloning and expression in *Escherichia coli* of the cDNA for murine tumor necrosis factor. *Proc Natl Acad Sci USA*

82: 6060–6064
11 Kriegler M, Perez C, DeFay K, Albert I, Lu SD (1988) A novel form of TNF/cachectin is a cell surface cytotoxic transmembrane protein: ramifications for the complex physiology of TNF. *Cell* 53: 45–53
12 Moss ML, Jin SL, Milla ME, Bickett DM, Burkhart W, Carter HL, Chen WJ, Clay WC, Didsbury JR, Hassler D et al (1997) Cloning of a disintegrin metalloproteinase that processes precursor tumour-necrosis factor-alpha. *Nature* 385: 733–736
13 Olsson I, Lantz M, Nilsson E, Peetre C, Thysell H, Grubb A, Adolf G (1989) Isolation and characterization of a tumor necrosis factor binding protein from urine. *Eur J Haematol* 42: 270–275
14 Seckinger P, Isaaz S, Dayer JM (1988) A human inhibitor of tumor necrosis factor alpha. *J Exp Med* 167: 1511–1516
15 Heim ME, Siegmund R, Illiger HJ, Klee M, Rieche K, Berdel WE, Edler L (1990) Tumor necrosis factor in advanced colorectal cancer: a phase II study. A trial of the phase I/II study group of the Association for Medical Oncology of the German Cancer Society. *Onkologie* 13: 444–447
16 Lenk H, Tanneberger S, Muller U, Ebert J, Shiga T (1989) Phase II clinical trial of high-dose recombinant human tumor necrosis factor. *Cancer Chemother Pharmacol* 24: 391–392
17 Locksley RM, Killeen N, Lenardo MJ (2001) The TNF and TNF receptor superfamilies: integrating mammalian biology. *Cell* 104: 487–501
18 Smith CA, Farrah T, Goodwin RG (1994) The TNF receptor superfamily of cellular and viral proteins: activation, costimulation, and death. *Cell* 76: 959–962
19 Wiley SR, Schooley K, Smolak PJ, Din WS, Huang CP, Nicholl JK, Sutherland GR, Smith TD, Rauch C, Smith CA et al (1995) Identification and characterization of a new member of the TNF family that induces apoptosis. *Immunity* 3: 673–682
20 Folks TM, Clouse KA, Justement J, Rabson A, Duh E, Kehrl JH, Fauci AS (1989) Tumor necrosis factor alpha induces expression of human immunodeficiency virus in a chronically infected T-cell clone. *Proc Natl Acad Sci USA* 86: 2365–2368
21 Tracey KJ, Fong Y, Hesse DG, Manogue KR, Lee AT, Kuo GC, Lowry SF, Cerami A (1987) Anti-cachectin/TNF monoclonal antibodies prevent septic shock during lethal bacteraemia. *Nature* 330: 662–664
22 Enbrel® (etanercept) [package insert]. Thousand Oaks, Calif. Amgen Inc. and Wyeth-Ayerst Pharmaceuticals, 2004
23 Remicade® (infliximab) [package insert]. Malvern, Pa. Centacor Inc., 2003
24 Humira® (adalimumab) [package insert]. North Chicago, Ill. Abbott Laboratories, 2003
25 Kaushansky K, Broudy VC, Harlan JM, Adamson JW (1988) Tumor necrosis factor-alpha and tumor necrosis factor-beta (lymphotoxin) stimulate the production of granulocyte-macrophage colony-stimulating factor, macrophage colony-stimulating factor, and IL-1 *in vivo*. *J Immunol* 141: 3410–3415
26 Smith CA, Davis T, Anderson D, Solam L, Beckmann MP, Jerzy R, Dower SK, Cosman D, Goodwin RG (1990) A receptor for tumor necrosis factor defines an unusual family of cellular and viral proteins. *Science* 248: 1019–1023
27 Jacobs CA, Sims JE, Mohler KM, Dower S, Giri JG, Smith CA, Mullarkey MF (1994) Soluble cytokine receptors as potential therapeutic antagonists. In: M Freund, H Link, RE Schmidt, K Welte, (eds): *Cytokines in Hemopoiesis, Oncology, and Immunology III*. Springer Verlag, Berlin, 453–460
28 Butler DM, Malfait AM, Mason LJ, Warden PJ, Kollias G, Maini RN, Feldmann M, Brennan FM (1997) DBA/1 mice expressing the human TNF-alpha transgene develop a severe, erosive arthritis: characterization of the cytokine cascade and cellular composition. *J Immunol* 159: 2867–2876
29 Alexopoulou L, Pasparakis M, Kollias G (1997) A murine transmembrane tumor necrosis factor (TNF) transgene induces arthritis by cooperative p55/p75 TNF receptor signaling. *Eur J Immunol* 27: 2588–2592
30 Piguet PF, Grau GE, Vesin C, Loetscher H, Gentz R, Lesslauer W (1992) Evolution of collagen arthritis in mice is arrested by treatment with anti-tumour necrosis factor (TNF) antibody or a recombinant soluble TNF receptor. *Immunology* 77: 510–514
31 Thorbecke GJ, Shah R, Leu CH, Kuruvilla AP, Hardison AM, Palladino MA (1992) Involvement of endogenous tumor necrosis factor alpha and transforming growth factor beta during induction of collagen type II arthritis in mice. *Proc Natl Acad Sci USA* 89: 7375–7379
32 Williams RO, Feldmann M, Maini RN (1992) Anti-tumor necrosis factor ameliorates joint disease in murine collagen-induced arthritis. *Proc Natl Acad Sci USA* 89: 9784–9788

33 Semmler J, Wachtel H, Endres S (1993) The specific type IV phosphodiesterase inhibitor rolipram suppresses tumor necrosis factor-alpha production by human mononuclear cells. *Int J Immunopharmacol* 15: 409–413
34 Sinha B, Semmler J, Eisenhut T, Eigler A, Endres S (1995) Enhanced tumor necrosis factor suppression and cyclic adenosine monophosphate accumulation by combination of phosphodiesterase inhibitors and prostanoids. *Eur J Immunol* 25: 147–153
35 Moreira AL, Sampaio EP, Zmuidzinas A, Frindt P, Smith KA, Kaplan G (1993) Thalidomide exerts its inhibitory action on tumor necrosis factor alpha by enhancing mRNA degradation. *J Exp Med* 177: 1675–1680
36 Aggarwal BB, Schwarz L, Hogan ME, Rando RF (1996) Triple helix-forming oligodeoxyribonucleotides targeted to the human tumor necrosis factor (TNF) gene inhibit TNF production and block the TNF-dependent growth of human glioblastoma tumor cells. *Cancer Res* 56: 5156–5164
37 Williams LM, Gibbons DL, Gearing A, Maini RN, Feldmann M, Brennan FM (1996) Paradoxical effects of a synthetic metalloproteinase inhibitor that blocks both p55 and p75 TNF receptor shedding and TNF alpha processing in RA synovial membrane cell cultures. *J Clin Invest* 97: 2833–2841
38 Kohno T, Stevens S, Louie J (2005) Adalimumab and infliximab bind to Fc-receptor and C1q and generate immunoprecipitation: A different mechanism from etanercept. [Abstract]. *J Am Acad Dermatol* 52: 36
39 Knight DM, Trinh H, Le J, Siegel S, Shealy D, McDonough M, Scallon B, Moore MA, Vilcek J, Daddona P et al (1993) Construction and initial characterization of a mouse-human chimeric anti-TNF antibody. *Mol Immunol* 30: 1443–1453
40 Lorenz HM, Antoni C, Valerius T, Repp R, Grunke M, Schwerdtner N, Nusslein H, Woody J, Kalden JR, Manger B (1996) *In vivo* blockade of TNF-alpha by intravenous infusion of a chimeric monoclonal TNF-alpha antibody in patients with rheumatoid arthritis. Short term cellular and molecular effects. *J Immunol* 156: 1646–1653
41 Scallon BJ, Moore MA, Trinh H, Knight DM, Ghrayeb J (1995) Chimeric anti-TNF-alpha monoclonal antibody cA2 binds recombinant transmembrane TNF-alpha and activates immune effector functions. *Cytokine* 7: 251–259
42 Elliott MJ, Maini RN, Feldmann M, Kalden JR, Antoni C, Smolen JS, Leeb B, Breedveld FC, Macfarlane JD, Bijl H et al (1994) Randomised double-blind comparison of chimeric monoclonal antibody to tumour necrosis factor alpha (cA2) *versus* placebo in rheumatoid arthritis. *Lancet* 344: 1105–1110
43 Moreland LW (1998) Soluble tumor necrosis factor receptor (p75) fusion protein (ENBREL) as a therapy for rheumatoid arthritis. *Rheum Dis Clin North Am* 24: 579–591
44 Targan SR, Hanauer SB, van Deventer SJ, Mayer L, Present DH, Braakman T, DeWoody KL, Schaible TF, Rutgeerts PJ (1997) A short-term study of chimeric monoclonal antibody cA2 to tumor necrosis factor alpha for Crohn's disease. Crohn's Disease cA2 Study Group. *N Engl J Med* 337: 1029–1035
45 Sandborn WJ, Hanauer SB, Katz S, Safdi M, Wolf DG, Baerg RD, Tremaine WJ, Johnson T, Diehl NN, Zinsmeister AR (2001) Etanercept for active Crohn's disease: a randomized, double-blind, placebo-controlled trial. *Gastroenterology* 121: 1088–1094
46 Dinarello CA (2005) Differences between anti-tumor necrosis factor-alpha monoclonal antibodies and soluble TNF receptors in host defense impairment. *J Rheumatol Suppl* 74: 40–47
47 Haraoui B, Keystone EC, Thorne JC, Pope JE, Chen I, Asare CG, Leff JA (2004) Clinical outcomes of patients with rheumatoid arthritis after switching from infliximab to etanercept. *J Rheumatol* 31: 2356–2359
48 van Vollenhoven RF (2004) Switching between biological agents. *Clin Exp Rheumatol* 22: S115–S121
49 Fisher CJ, Jr, Agosti JM, Opal SM, Lowry SF, Balk RA, Sadoff JC, Abraham E, Schein RM, Benjamin E (1996) Treatment of septic shock with the tumor necrosis factor receptor:Fc fusion protein. The Soluble TNF Receptor Sepsis Study Group. *N Engl J Med* 334: 1697–1702
50 Davis JC, Jr, Van Der Heijde D, Braun J, Dougados M, Cush J, Clegg DO, Kivitz A, Fleischmann R, Inman R, Tsuji W (2003) Recombinant human tumor necrosis factor receptor (etanercept) for treating ankylosing spondylitis: a randomized, controlled trial. *Arthritis Rheum* 48: 3230–3236
51 Gottlieb AB, Matheson RT, Lowe N, Krueger GG, Kang S, Goffe BS, Gaspari AA, Ling M, Weinstein GD, Nayak A et al (2003) A randomized trial of etanercept as monotherapy for psoriasis. *Arch Dermatol* 139: 1627–1632; discussion 1632

52 Klareskog L, van der Heijde D, de Jager JP, Gough A, Kalden J, Malaise M, Martin Mola E, Pavelka K, Sany J, Settas L et al (2004) Therapeutic effect of the combination of etanercept and methotrexate compared with each treatment alone in patients with rheumatoid arthritis: double-blind randomised controlled trial. *Lancet* 363: 675–681

53 Lovell DJ, Giannini EH, Reiff A, Cawkwell GD, Silverman ED, Nocton JJ, Stein LD, Gedalia A, Ilowite NT, Wallace CA et al (2000) Etanercept in children with polyarticular juvenile rheumatoid arthritis. Pediatric Rheumatology Collaborative Study Group. *N Engl J Med* 342: 763–769

54 Mease PJ, Kivitz AJ, Burch FX, Siegel EL, Cohen SB, Ory P, Salonen D, Rubenstein J, Sharp JT, Tsuji W (2004) Etanercept treatment of psoriatic arthritis: safety, efficacy, and effect on disease progression. *Arthritis Rheum* 50: 2264–2272

55 Clinical Trials.gov Web Site (Accessed March 28, 2005) *Onercept in the Treatment and Re-Treatment of Subjects with Moderate to Severe Plaque Psoriasis.* At: http://www.clinicaltrials.gov/ct/gui/show/NCT00090129?order=1

56 Furst DE, Weisman M, Paulus HE, Bulpitt K, Weinblatt M, Polisson R, Zaug M, Kneer J, Van der Auwera P, Stevens RM (2003) Intravenous human recombinant tumor necrosis factor receptor p55-Fc IgG1 fusion protein, Ro 45-2081 (lenercept): results of a dose-finding study in rheumatoid arthritis. *J Rheumatol* 30: 2123–2126

57 Lesslauer W, Tabuchi H, Gentz R, Brockhaus M, Schlaeger EJ, Grau G, Piguet PF, Pointaire P, Vassalli P, Loetscher H (1991) Recombinant soluble tumor necrosis factor receptor proteins protect mice from lipopolysaccharide-induced lethality. *Eur J Immunol* 21: 2883–2886

58 Fernandez-Botran R (2000) Soluble cytokine receptors: novel immunotherapeutic agents. *Expert Opin Investig Drugs* 9: 497–514

59 Moreland L, Gugliotti R, King K, Chase W, Weisman M, Greco T, Fife R, Korn J, Simms R, Tesser J et al (2001) Results of a phase-I/II randomized, masked, placebo-controlled trial of recombinant human interleukin-11 (rhIL-11) in the treatment of subjects with active rheumatoid arthritis. *Arthritis Res* 3: 247–252

60 Asadullah K, Docke WD, Ebeling M, Friedrich M, Belbe G, Audring H, Volk HD, Sterry W (1999) Interleukin 10 treatment of psoriasis: clinical results of a phase 2 trial. *Arch Dermatol* 135: 187–192

61 Trepicchio WL, Ozawa M, Walters IB, Kikuchi T, Gilleaudeau P, Bliss JL, Schwertschlag U, Dorner AJ, Krueger JG (1999) Interleukin-11 therapy selectively downregulates type I cytokine proinflammatory pathways in psoriasis lesions. *J Clin Invest* 104: 1527–1537

62 Stevens SR, Hanifin JM, Hamilton T, Tofte SJ, Cooper KD (1998) Long-term effectiveness and safety of recombinant human interferon gamma therapy for atopic dermatitis despite unchanged serum IgE levels. *Arch Dermatol* 134: 799–804

63 Panitch H, Miller A, Paty D, Weinshenker B (2004) Interferon beta-1b in secondary progressive MS: results from a 3-year controlled study. *Neurology* 63: 1788–1795

64 Arend WP (2002) The balance between IL-1 and IL-1Ra in disease. *Cytokine Growth Factor Rev* 13: 323–340

65 Dinarello CA, Cannon JG, Wolff SM, Bernheim HA, Beutler B, Cerami A, Figari IS, Palladino MA, Jr, O'Connor JV (1986) Tumor necrosis factor (cachectin) is an endogenous pyrogen and induces production of interleukin 1. *J Exp Med* 163: 1433–1450

66 Horai R, Saijo S, Tanioka H, Nakae S, Sudo K, Okahara A, Ikuse T, Asano M, Iwakura Y (2000) Development of chronic inflammatory arthropathy resembling rheumatoid arthritis in interleukin 1 receptor antagonist-deficient mice. *J Exp Med* 191: 313–320

67 van den Berg WB, Joosten LA, van de Loo FA (1999) TNF alpha and IL-1 beta are separate targets in chronic arthritis. *Clin Exp Rheumatol* 17: S105–S114

68 Kineret® (anakinra) [package insert]. Thousand Oaks, Calif. Amgen Inc., 2002

69 Beck JT, Hsu SM, Wijdenes J, Bataille R, Klein B, Vesole D, Hayden K, Jagannath S, Barlogie B (1994) Brief report: alleviation of systemic manifestations of Castleman's disease by monoclonal anti-interleukin-6 antibody. *N Engl J Med* 330: 602–605

70 Gringeri A, Santagostino E, Cusini M, Muca-Perja M, Marinoni A, Mannucci PM, Burny A, Criscuolo M, Lu W, Andrieu JM et al (1996) Absence of clinical, virological, and immunological signs of progression in HIV-1-infected patients receiving active anti-interferon-alpha immunization: a 30-month follow-up report. *J Acquir Immune Defic Syndr Hum Retrovirol* 13: 55–67

71 Hart TK, Blackburn MN, Brigham-Burke M, Dede K, Al-Mahdi N, Zia-Amirhosseini P, Cook RM (2002) Preclinical efficacy and safety of pascolizumab (SB 240683): a humanized anti-interleukin-4 antibody with therapeutic potential in asthma. *Clin Exp Immunol* 130: 93–100

72 Leckie MJ, ten Brinke A, Khan J, Diamant Z, O'Connor BJ, Walls CM, Mathur AK, Cowley HC, Chung KF, Djukanovic R et al (2000) Effects of an interleukin-5 blocking monoclonal antibody on eosinophils, airway hyper-responsiveness, and the late asthmatic response. *Lancet* 356: 2144–2148

73 Llorente L, Richaud-Patin Y, Garcia-Padilla C, Claret E, Jakez-Ocampo J, Cardiel MH, Alcocer-Varela J, Grangeot-Keros L, Alarcon-Segovia D, Wijdenes J et al (2000) Clinical and biologic effects of anti-interleukin-10 monoclonal antibody administration in systemic lupus erythematosus. *Arthritis Rheum* 43: 1790–1800

74 Lodolce JP, Burkett PR, Koka RM, Boone DL, Ma A (2002) Regulation of lymphoid homeostasis by interleukin-15. *Cytokine Growth Factor Rev* 13: 429–439

75 Plater-Zyberk C, Joosten LA, Helsen MM, Sattonnet-Roche P, Siegfried C, Alouani S, van De Loo FA, Graber P, Aloni S, Cirillo R et al (2001) Therapeutic effect of neutralizing endogenous IL-18 activity in the collagen-induced model of arthritis. *J Clin Invest* 108: 1825–1832

76 St Clair EW, van der Heijde DM, Smolen JS, Maini RN, Bathon JM, Emery P, Keystone E, Schiff M, Kalden JR, Wang B et al (2004) Combination of infliximab and methotrexate therapy for early rheumatoid arthritis: a randomized, controlled trial. *Arthritis Rheum* 50: 3432–3443

77 van der Heijde D, Dijkmans B, Geusens P, Sieper J, DeWoody K, Williamson P, Braun J (2005) Efficacy and safety of infliximab in patients with ankylosing spondylitis: results of a randomized, placebo-controlled trial (ASSERT). *Arthritis Rheum* 52: 582–591

78 Weinblatt ME, Keystone EC, Furst DE, Moreland LW, Weisman MH, Birbara CA, Teoh LA, Fischkoff SA, Chartash EK (2003) Adalimumab, a fully human anti-tumor necrosis factor alpha monoclonal antibody, for the treatment of rheumatoid arthritis in patients taking concomitant methotrexate: the ARMADA trial. *Arthritis Rheum* 48: 35–45

79 Choy EH, Hazleman B, Smith M, Moss K, Lisi L, Scott DG, Patel J, Sopwith M, Isenberg DA (2002) Efficacy of a novel PEGylated humanized anti-TNF fragment (CDP870) in patients with rheumatoid arthritis: a phase II double-blinded, randomized, dose-escalating trial. *Rheumatology (Oxford)* 41: 1133–1137

TNF-alpha Inhibitors
Edited by Jeffrey M. Weinberg and Robin Buchholz

Pharmacology of TNF inhibitors

Rahul Shukla and Ronald B. Vender

McMaster University and Dermatrials Research, Hamilton, Ontario, Canada

Tumor necrosis factor family

The tumor necrosis factor (TNF) superfamily of cytokines activate signaling pathways for cell survival, death, and differentiation that orchestrate the development, organization and homeostasis of lymphoid, mammary, neuronal and ectodermal tissues [1]. The TNF superfamily of proteins includes soluble cytokines and membrane proteins that share sequence homologies and fold into homotrimeric triangular pyramids that bind to structurally similar receptors [2]. A number of proteins comprise the TNF family including TNF alpha (TNF-α) and lymphotoxin (previously termed TNF beta), members of the TNF family which are particular important in T cell effector function. The trimeric structure characteristic of all members of the TNF family, and the ligand-induced trimerization of their receptors seems to be the critical event mediating the effects of TNF proteins [2]. The pleiotropic effects of TNFs in immune and inflammatory responses implicate them as an important mediatory in many diseases [3].

Lymphotoxin

Lymphotoxin alpha (LT-α) is a multifunctional cytokine structurally homologous to TNF-α [4, 5], which is expressed by activated lymphocytes [6] as a soluble homotrimer or membrane-associated heterotrimer with LT beta [7]. In its soluble form LT-α can bind with equal affinity to either TNF receptor I (TNFR1, also known as p55) or TNF receptor II (TNFRII, also known as p75) [9]. The membrane bound form of LT-α occurs through the formation of a heterotrimer with LT-β, a membrane-bound TNF protein. The complexed LT-α and LT-β form LTa1β2, a heterotrimer that does not bind to TNFR I or II, but instead signals exclusively through the LT-β receptor (LTβR) [9]. The LTa1β2–LTβR interaction is believed to play an essential role in secondary lymphoid organ development and function [10]. Furthermore, the action of LTa1β2 is believed to be critical in lymphoid organogenesis and paramount in the differentiation of Va14*i* natural killer T (NKT) cells, a lymphocyte subset with important immunoregulatory properties [10].

Lymphotoxin in disease

LT-α shares similar properties to TNF-α such as the activation of T and B lymphocytes and inducing the release of inflammatory cytokines from fibroblasts and endothelial cells. These effects are believed to occur after binding of LT-α to either TNFR1 or TNFR2 [11]. In comparison to TNF-α, the role of LT-α in disease processes is not well defined. Although LT-α is believed to play a role in psoriasis [12], further evidence is required to clearly define LT-α role in rheumatoid arthritis (RA) despite the presence of elevated levels of LT-α in the synovial joints of patients suffering from RA [11]. A definitive role for LT-α in psoriatic arthritis has not been established either; therefore, the significance of LT-α in psoriatic arthritis also remains unclear [13].

TNF-α

TNF-α is a homotrimeric proinflammatory cytokine activated by mainly macrophages and T lymphocytes during acute inflammation. TNF-α exists in both transmembrane and soluble forms. The 26 kDa membrane-bound form of TNF-α is cleaved by TNF-α converting enzyme (TACE) to release a 17 kDa soluble circulating form [14, 15].

Although both forms of TNF-α are functional, the soluble form is thought to be more active and interacts with TNFRI and TNFRII to exert its action [16]. Both TNFRI and TNFRII are bound to the surface of cells such as macrophages, lympocytes, keratinocytes, and endothelial cells. After TNF-α binds to either TNFRI or TNFRII it facilitates the movement of the nuclear transcription factor NF-kappaB into the nucleus where it induces the transcription of genes producing cytokines contributing to the inflammatory cascade [17, 18].

In addition to membrane bound receptors for TNF-α, soluble receptors such as p75 also naturally exist which seem to act as competitive inhibitors for TNF-α binding to cell surface receptors [19, 20]. The activity and amount of these receptors, however, are not sufficient enough to block the inflammatory cascade caused by TNF-α in disease states [20, 21].

TNF-α in disease

TNF-α is known to play a crucial role in the pathogenesis of many chronic inflammatory diseases. Elevated levels of TNF-α have been demonstrated in Crohn's disease (CD), psoriasis, psoriatic arthritis and RA suggesting a role for TNF-α in their pathogenesis [11, 22–24]. Although TNF-α plays a critical role in the activation of innate and acquired immune responses, the persistence of the immune response and inappropriate production of TNF-α can produce pathological changes resulting from chronic inflammation and tissue damage

Table 1. Effects of excessive TNF-α production on various cell types

Cell type	Action of TNF-α	Effect
Macrophage	Increased proinflammatory cytokine production Increased chemokine production	Increased inflammation Swelling of joints
Keratinocyte	Increased proliferation	Scale and thickness
Endothelial	Increased expression of adhesion molecules Increased production of VEGF	Increased leukocyte infiltration into skin and joints Increased angiogenesis and erythema Auspitz sign
Hepatocyte	Increased acute phase response	Increased C-reactive protein
Synoviocyte (fibroblast-like)	Increased metalloproteinase synthesis	Articular cartilage degradation
T lymphocyte	Increased proinflammatory cytokine production Increased nuclear transcription factor activation T cell activation	Increased inflammation
Dendritic cell	Increased proinflammatory cytokine production Dendritic cell maturation Increased dendritic cell migration from skin to lymph nodes T cell activation and differentiation	Increased inflammation

VEGF, vascular endothelial growth factor.
Reprinted from Journal of the American Academy of Dermatology, 49(2 Suppl), Goffe B, Cather JC. Etanercept: An overview. S105-11, c (2003), with permission from Elsevier Inc.

[25]. Refer to Table 1 for the effects of excessive TNF-α production on various cell types [25].

In the skin, the presence of TNF-α promotes proliferation and reduces keratinocyte destruction resulting in hyperproliferation of the epidermis. TNF-α within the dermis acts to recruit macrophages to the area and induces the secretion of proinflammatory cytokines and chemokines [26]. Increased levels of TNF-α within the skin act to increase levels of interleukin (IL) 6, IL8, IL1; cytokines which act to promote hyperproliferation of keratinocytes. A reduction in keratinocyte apoptosis and cell cycling mediated by TNF-α also act to contribute to a state of hyperproliferation by diminishing keratinocyte destruction [27].

Further evidence implicating TNF-α as part of pathogenic process in inflammatory skin conditions is suggested from findings that demonstrate elevations of TACE mRNA in psoriatic lesions [15]. TACE is a metalloproteinase that acts to cleave the extracellular domain of membrane bound TNF-α releasing the soluble form of the cytokine. Increased levels of TACE in psoriatic lesions are primarily believed to be the result of increased mast cell production of TNF-α [15]. Elevated levels of TACE, therefore, act as a source of TNF-α potentially contributing to the pathogenic process of psoriasis.

TNF-α has also been cited to mediate key processes in inflammatory joint destruction. Specifically, TNF-α induces prostaglandin E2 and leukotriene synthesis, molecules known to incite bone resorption and cartilage degradation in arthritis [28, 29]. Further joint destruction occurs through the synergistic action of TNF-α and IL1, cytokines which act in concert to produce matrix metalloproteinase, a class of zinc dependent peptidases participating in extracellular degradation and remodeling [30].

Maintenance of the abnormal inflammatory response in the skin and joints occurs from the TNF-α-induced expression of adhesion molecules and production of vascular endothelial growth factor (VEGF), substances that act to facilitate the migration of inflammatory cytokines and which encourage angiogenesis, respectively [26].

A role of TNF-α has been suggested in CD, as well. Defective T cell apoptosis appears to play a role in the development of inflammation in patients with CD [31]. The uncontrolled proliferation of activated lamina propia lymphocytes that results from defects in apoptosis is expected to contribute to chronic mucosal inflammation and an excess of proinflammatory cytokines such as TNF-α [22]. In addition to the development of inflammatory molecules, TNF-α has a role in mucosal barrier dysfunction in the gut of patients with inflammatory processes such as CD [32].

Pharmacological intervention against TNF-α

Evidence that the proinflammatory cytokine TNF-α plays a major role in the development and maintenance of diseases such as CD, psoriasis, psoriatic arthritis and RA provides a rationale for the use of anti-TNF-α therapies. Currently, there are two classes of drugs that reduce TNF bioavailability: soluble TNF receptors (etanercept) and TNF-binding monoclonal antibodies (infliximab and adalimumab). By blocking the activity of TNF-α these drugs have an ameliorable effect when managing diseases where TNF-α is inappropriately elevated. The pharmacology of these drugs will be examined in the following section.

Structure

Soluble TNF receptor

Etanercept

Etanercept is a human fusion protein formed by the fusion of two soluble domains of the human p75 TNF-receptor to the Fc portion of the type 1 human immunoglobulin (IgG1) [33]. In addition to binding to both membrane-bound and soluble forms of TNF-α, etanercept binds to LT-α, thereby inhibiting the biologic effects of both of these mediators [11, 33]. Etanercept is produced by recombinant DNA technology in a Chinese Hamster Ovary (CHO) mammalian cell expression system and consists of 934 amino acids with an approximate weight of approximately 150 kDa [25, 33]. Refer to Figure 1 for a schematic drawing of etanercept.

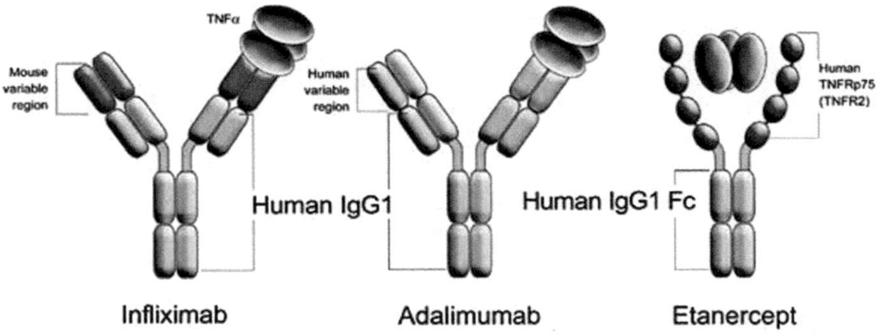

Figure 1. Anti-TNF molecules bind to and neutralize the activity of TNFα. Infliximab and adalimumab are monoclonal antibodies. Infliximab is a mouse/human chimera that joints the variable regions of a mouse antibody to the constant region of human IgG1, and adalimumab is a human IgG1 antibody. Etanercept is a dimeric fusion protein that joins the human p75 TNF receptor to the Fc domain of human IgG1. Reprinted from *Seminars in Arthritis and Rheumatism*, 34(suppl. 1), Anderson PJ. Tumor necrosis factor inhibitors clinical implications of their different immunogenicity profiles. 19–22, 2005, with permission from Elsevier Inc.

TNF binding monoclonal antibodies

Adalimumab

Adalimumab is a recombinant IgG1 monoclonal antibody composed of two kappa light chains and two IgG1 heavy chains. Created using phage display technology, adalimumab is comprised of fully human heavy and light chain variable regions and human IgG1 heavy chain and kappa light sequences, resulting in a molecule that is indistinguishable from human IgG1 [34]. Although adalimumab does bind to both soluble and membrane forms of TNF [35], it does not bind to or neutralize LT-α [36].

Adalimumab consists of 1,330 amino acids and has a molecular weight of approximately 148 kDa [36]. It is produced by recombinant DNA technology in a mammalian expression system and is purified by a process that includes specific viral inactivation and removal steps. Refer to Figure 1 for a schematic drawing of adalimumab.

Infliximab

Infliximab is a chimeric anti-TNF-α monoclonal antibody produced by joining the human IgG1 constant region to a murine derived antigen binding variable region [37]. Infliximab has binding specificity for soluble and membranous TNF-α and does not bind with or inhibit receptor mediated activity of LT-α [26].

Infliximab has a molecular weight of 149 kDa and is produced by recombinant cell line cultured by continuous perfusion [38]. A series of steps are taken, which includes measures to inactivate and remove viruses, to purify infliximab [38]. Refer to Figure 1 for a schematic drawing of infliximab.

Binding characteristics

Monoclonal antibodies are believed to be relatively dynamic in comparison to etanercept in terms of immune complex formation as they have been suggested to have the potential to form a greater number of immune complexes. As a result of the trimeric structure of TNF-α and the bivalent nature of antibodies such as adalimumab and infliximab, a variety of immune complexes may form including the cross-linking of several IgGs [40]. In contrast, TNF:Fc fusion molecules are believed to be more restricted as a result steric hindrance, preventing cross-linking of multiple TNF-α trimers [40].

The potential to form an array of immune complexes increases the probability of forming a relatively large immune complex, which may rapidly clear from the body. Adalimumab, for instance, is believed to form a number of immune complexes of varying weight which eventually result in the formation of a thermally stable molecule consisting of a circular chain of three alternating adalimumab and TNF-α molecules that weighs approximately 598 kD. An immune complex of such weight would be expected to clear from the body very rapidly, thus making adalimumab a very efficient molecule for binding and removing TNF-α from the circulation [29].

Although mechanisms of immunoprecipitation may differ between monoclonal antibodies and soluble receptors, binding affinity is similar for adalimumab, etanercept and infliximab. Affinity is the strength of a reversible, monovalent association between an antibody and antigen. Affinity is expressed in molar units as the antigen dissociation constant, K_D, where smaller values of K_D reflect a greater affinity. Since affinity is a primary determinant of the concentration of antibody required to bind a given fraction of antigen it is often an important determinant of the therapeutic dose [41].

Adalimumab has been reported to bind with TNF-α with a relatively high affinity where studies have reported K_D values ranging from 7.05×10^{-11} M [42] to 1.0×10^{-10} M [39]. Although both etanercept and infliximab also bind to TNF-α avidly, controversy exists in the literature as to which therapeutic protein binds to TNF-α with greater affinity. Scallon and colleagues suggest that infliximab has a slightly lower K_D of 4.5×10^{-10} M, compared with 1.15×10^{-9} M for etanercept [43]. The larger affinity for TNF-α displayed by infliximab is believed to be a consequence of the greater stability of the TNF-α/infliximab complex [43].

Conversely, data has also demonstrated a greater affinity of etanercept for TNF-α, when compared to infliximab. According to Smith and colleagues K_D values of 2.35×10^{-11} M and 1.17×10^{-10} M were obtained for etanercept and infliximab, respectively [44]. The greater affinity of etanercept was credited to the faster rate of ligand binding [44].

Further investigations examining the binding characteristics of both infliximab and etanercept may prove valuable in conclusively determining K_D values for each drug.

Immunogenicity

All biologic TNF-α inhibitors are foreign proteins and therefore potentially immunogenic [45]. Potential clinical effects arising from immunogenicity gives rise to pathological concerns including the occurrence of severe allergic or anaphylactic responses or an immune response that could induce autoimmunity to the patient's own endogenous protein [45, 46]. From a pharmacological perspective, an immune response to a therapeutic protein may impair targeting of therapeutic antibodies and accelerate clearance and reduce serum levels of antibody products [47, 48].

Etanercept has been shown to have a low rate of immunogenicity when studied in patients with psoriasis, RA and congestive heart failure (CHF). Incidences of anti-etanercept antibodies were observed to be 2%, 0.6% and 0% in clinical trials of patients with RA, CHF and psoriasis, respectively [49, 50].

The importance of using appropriate assays when studying the immunogenicity of etanercept has been underlined by the varying rates of immunogenicity that result from using different assay configurations [49].

Structural differences in therapeutic proteins are a major factor contributing to a drug's immunogenicity and should be examined when comparing the immunogenicity of therapeutic proteins. As a result of its compositional resemblance to human IgG1 and because it contains no non-human sequences, adalimumab may have a reduced immunogenicity when compared to infliximab or etanercept [51]. Clinical evidence appears to corroborate with theoretical ideologies as pooled cumulative incidence of anti-adalimumab antibody formation is relatively low when compared to infliximab [52]. The incidence of antibody formation ranged from 8–68% across studies in patients receiving infliximab while values ranging from 6–12% were found in patients receiving adalimumab [52, 53]. Concomitant therapy with methotrexate was associated with reduced incidence of antibody formation to both drugs.

When examining data on the immunogenicity of adalimumab and infliximab from pooled results one must be cognoscente of the limitations that prevent an investigator from making a direct comparison. Differences in patient populations (RA *versus* Crohn's disease) across studies and the possible lack of standardization in the assay methods used (double-capture enzyme-linked immunosorbent assay) [52] are factors that make comparing immunogenicity profiles of therapeutic proteins difficult.

Pharmacokinetics

Conceptual model of TNF factor inhibitor pharmacokinetics and pharmacodynamics

The therapeutic goal when administering TNF-α antagonists is to eliminate the surplus of TNF-α in the blood and from sites of inflammation [54]. Reductions should be made such that TNF-α values do not fall below levels that may comprise an individual's immunocompetency.

Nestorov described a conceptual model outlining the interactions that occur from TNF-α factor antagonist administration to the clinical response produced by the drug outlined in Figure 2 [54]. TNF-α acts as a ligand for TNF-α antagonists and is synthesized and expressed by immune cells throughout tissue/fluids of the body. Once TNF antagonist is administered and absorped from the site of administration, a number of interactions occur between tissues/fluids and blood. These interactions describe the pharmacokinetics of a drug. Upon reaching the target site TNF antagonists bind to soluble TNFs and TNF expressed on the surface of various cells triggering the pharmacologic mechanism of action; a process described as the pharmacodynamics of the drug. Nestorov's model demonstrates that pharmacokinetics of a drug precedes the

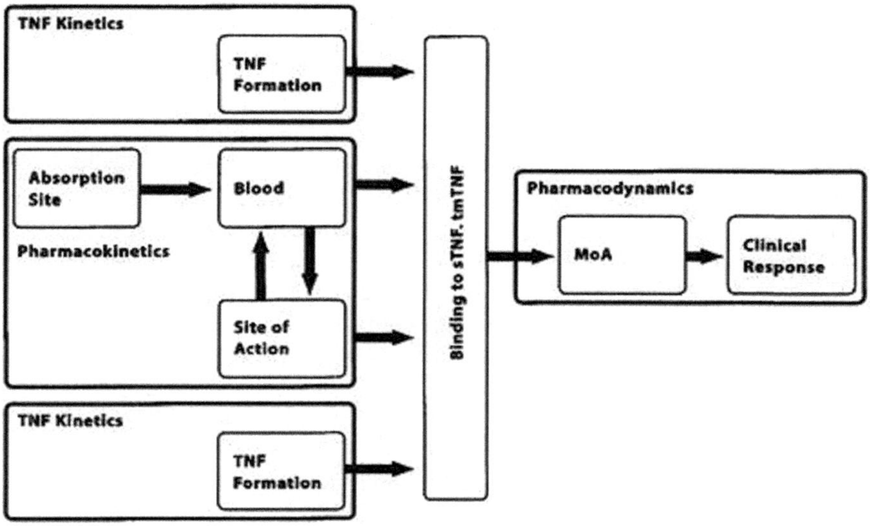

Figure 2. Cascade of processes after administration of TNF antagonists. sTNF: soluble tumor necrosis factor; MoA: pharmacologic mechanisms of action; tmTNF: transmembrane TNF. Reprinted from *The Journal of Rheumatology*, 74, Nestorov I. Clinical pharmacokinetics of tumor necrosis factor antagonists. 13–18, 2005, with permission from the Journal of Rheumatology.

therapeutic action and should be examined when differentiating between drugs producing a similar response [54].

Administration and absorption

The majority of FDA-approved therapeutic proteins are administered intravenously or subcutaneously. Intravenous (IV) administration is often preferred because it circumvents presystemic degradation, allows for complete systemic availability and rapid delivery of proteins to systemic circulation and achievement of high concentrations [55]. Intravenous administration also has its drawbacks. In addition to lack of convenience, it may also not provide an optimal concentration–time profile.

Dosing regimens that lead to smooth concentration–time profiles are preferred to acute dosage regimens yielding large peak-to-trough concentration ratios at steady state [54]. Drugs administered intravenously as a bolus or constant rate infusion may cause acute concentration-time profiles with high peaks and low minimums, particularly if loading and maintenance doses are large. Extreme concentrations may bind excessive TNF-α and consequently, lower an organism's defense against potential infection [54]. Conversely, low minimums may lead to concentrations of a drug that are subtherapeutic.

Infliximab is administered by 2 h intravenous infusion using a combination of a loading dosing scheme (weeks 0, 2 and 6) and a uniform maintenance dosing scheme with a dosing period of 4–8 weeks [56]. Maximum serum concentrations of 165 ± 42 mg/mL have been reported for infliximab in psoriasis patients receiving 5 mg/kg measured post second infusion [56, 57]. An average serum value of 27.0 mg/mL was present in psoriasis patients following a 5 mg/kg infusion, during the first 26 weeks of a dosing regimen consisting of infusions at 0, 2 and 6 weeks [56, 57]. Reported minimum concentration values in psoriasis patients following doses at weeks 0, 2 and 6 have been reported to be 8.3 ± 11.9 mg/mL [56, 57]. Although data for the steady-state pharmacokinetics is limited, a number of references indicate that no further accumulation of the drug is observed with doses of 3–10 mg/kg after the loading period with infusions at weeks 0, 2, and 6 [57–60].

As a result of significant loading doses (630–2,100 mg delivered within 6 weeks for a 70 kg individual) and fairly high maintenance doses for infliximab (210 mg to 700 mg for 70 kg individual), a situation may result where acute concentration–time profiles with very high peaks and low minimums are created [56]. Significant flux in drug concentration may predispose and individual to infection if drug concentrations are excessive or may lead to poor efficacy if the serum concentrations of the therapeutic molecule are too low.

Both etanercept and adalimumab are administered via subcutaneous (SC) injection and are absorbed slowly. Although absorbed more slowly through the SC route of administration drugs injected in this fashion may result in a more uniform concentration–time profile; especially if the agents are eliminated slowly and have moderate maintenance doses. Etanercept is administered by a quasi-form (BIW) or uniform (qW) multiple dosing regimen with a dosing period of 1 week while adalimumab is administered by a multiple dosing regimen with a dosing period of 1 or every 2 weeks [54].

Subcutaneous administration of therapeutic proteins may result in the molecule either entering the systemic circulation via blood capillaries or through lymphatic vessels [61]. There appears to be a linear relationship between the molecular weight of a biologic agent and the proportion of the dose absorbed by the lymphatics. Macromolecules larger than 16 kDa are absorbed primarily into lymphatic vessels while those under 1 kDa are mostly absorbed in the blood capillaries [62].

Etanercept and adalimumab are molecules sharing molecular weights of approximately 150 kDa and are therefore, predominantly absorbed into lymphatic vessels. As lymph fluid drains into the vascular system, the absorption of drugs continues for hours. The maximum serum concentration of etanercept in psoriasis patients receiving 50 mg biweekly injections was reported to be 4.90 ± 2.5 mg/L, 69 ± 48 h following injection [56]. In addition, psoriasis patients receiving the same dosing regimen were found to have an average serum concentration of 3.67 ± 2.0 mg/mL and a minimum concentration of 1.21 ± 0.7 mg/mL [56].

Concentration profiles of psoriasis patients receiving adalimumab have not been published as of yet. However, various concentration parameters have been reported for RA patients receiving adalimumab. After a time period of 90 ± 48 h following a dosing regimen consisting of 40 mg injection every other week, RA patients were found to have a peak serum concentration of 7.7 ± 3.4 mg/mL [56, 62]. Average and minimum serum concentration values of 5.5 ± 2.5 mg/mL and 3.8 ± 2.1 mg/mL have also been reported in patients receiving the same dosing regimen, respectively [56, 62].

Pharmacokinetic information for adalimumab and etanercept reveals that a uniform concentration–time profile is maintained when either of these drugs is administered. The combination of slow absorption rates following SC administration, slow elimination rates and appropriate dosing frequencies are factors which help to produce steady concentration–time profile for both drugs [62].

The extent of absorption of therapeutic proteins may vary depending on the extent of presystemic antibody degradation by proteolytic enzymes [64]. In general, most investigations of antibody or therapeutic protein following subcutaneous or intramuscular dosing have reported bioavailabilities ranging from 50–100% [65–68]. Bioavailabilities observed for both adalimumab and etanercept are in accord with this trend. After a 40 mg subcutaneous dose of adalimumab an average absolute bioavailability was found to be 64% while a mean absolute bioavailability of 58% was observed for etanercept, following a 10 mg subcutaneous administration [36, 68].

Unlike conventional small molecule drugs, proteins are generally not therapeutically active upon oral administration [69–71]. Low systemic bioavailability often results after oral administration because of the proteolytic activity of the enzymes found within the gastrointestinal tract and by degradation that occurs in the acidic environment of the stomach [72]. Bioavailability is further reduced by gastrointestinal mucosa, which presents a major absorption barrier for water soluble molecules like peptides and proteins [71].

Volume of distribution

The pharmacokinetic property that characterizes drug distribution is the volume of distribution at steady state [54]. The volume of distribution of a drug is determined largely by its physiochemical properties – such as charge and lipophilicity – protein binding, and its dependency on active transport processes [72]. As a result of their large size, the apparent volume of distribution of therapeutic proteins is usually small, and limited to the volume of extracellular space due to their limited mobility secondary to impaired passage through biomembranes [73, 74].

Infliximab has a volume of distribution of 3–5 litres (L) [54]. The volume of distribution at steady state is primarily within the vascular compartment and distributes little outside the blood circulation into inflamed tissues. The volume of distribution increases slightly for adalimumab, with values ranging from 4.7–6.0 L [36]. In comparison to infliximab and adalimumab, etanercept has the greatest volume of distribution at steady state with a value of 12 ± 6 L [75]. The extent of extravascular distribution of etanercept, however, is still expected to be very small [76]. Analysis of TNF antagonist binding outside the serum as well as generation of data for concentration profiles of drugs in various target tissues will help clarify the meaning and effect of the observed differences in volume of distribution [54]. Although little data has been gathered on concentration time profiles of TNF antagonists outside the serum, a clinical trial consisting of five RA patients has demonstrated adalimumab concentrations in synovial fluid ranging from 31–96% of those in the serum [36].

Elimination

Conclusive evidence outlining the precise method of elimination for adalimumab, etanercept and infliximab remains to be elucidated. Currently, it is assumed that following binding of etanercept to TNF-α, the complex is metabolized through a peptide and amino acid pathway with either recycling of amino acids or elimination in bile and urine [75]. A clearance rate of 160 ± 80 mL/h and half life of 4.25 ± 1.25 days have been observed for etanercept [33]. The Fc portion of IgG1 serves to stabilize etanercept and cause a three-fold increase in the drug's half-life [19, 77].

Although no formal studies have been conducted to date to evaluate the metabolism of and excretion of adalimumab, it is expected that its metabolism and excretion would follow the course of other IgG molecules as adalimumab is an IgG1 antibody of entirely human sequences [36]. One may expect infliximab to be metabolized and eliminated in similar fashion, despite infliximab's murine variable regions.

The vast majority of immunoglobulin is expected to be eliminated by catabolism. Immunoglobulins are believed to be primarily metabolized within sites that are in rapid equilibrium with the plasma; however, the exact anatomical locations of antibody catabolism remain to be identified [78].

Unlike information regarding the modes of elimination for adalimumab and infliximab, data regarding the half lives of both drugs has been observed and reported. According to several single dose studies with values of intravenously administered adalimumab ranging from 0.25–10.0 mg/kg, the mean terminal half-life was approximated to be 14 days with values ranging 10–20 days across studies [36]. The systemic clearance of adalimumab was also estimated from these single dose studies and was found to be 12 ml/h [36]. Increased clearance rates of adalimumab have been observed in patients who develop antibodies to the drug while decreased clearance rates have been reported in patients from 40–75 years old [36].

Infliximab is thought to have a shorter median terminal half-life than adalimumab ranging from 8.0–9.5 days after administration of 3 mg/kg to

10 mg/kg doses to patients with RA and 5 mg/kg in Crohn's disease [38]. The generation of anti-infliximab antibodies has been demonstrated to further reduce the half-life of infliximab. In RA patients receiving infliximab between 1 and 6 months following their initial treatment, the terminal half-life of antibody positive patents was 48 h compared to 190 h for antibody negative patients [79]. Though the clearance of the drug is unknown [80], systemic accumulation does not occur after continued repeated treatment with 3 mg/kg or 10 mg/kg at 4 or 8 week intervals [38].

The relatively long half-lives demonstrated by the monoclonal antibodies adalimumab and infliximab can be explained their structural similarity to human IgG; an immunoglobulin with an extraordinarily long half-life. The prolonged half-life demonstrated by human IgG is due to catabolic protection by neonatal Fc receptor (FcRn), a protein that promotes IgG absorption and protection from systemic elimination. FcRn is expressed on hepatocytes, endothelial cells, and phagocytic cells of the reticuloendothelial cell system [81]. When the IgG undergoes endocytosis, the low pH of the endosome promotes binding of the IgG Fc domain to FcRn, which recycles IgG to the cell surface and salvages IgG from lysosomal degradation [82, 83]. Unbound IgG proceeds to the lysosome and undergoes proteolytic degradation [55].

Pharmacodynamics

Soluble TNF receptor

Etanercept

In order for TNF-α mediated events to occur, binding to TNFR1 and TNFR2, multimerization of these receptors, and subsequent signal transduction through the receptors intracellular domains is required [84, 85]. LT-α binds also binds to TNFRI and TNFR2 and can also initiate inflammatory processes similar to TNF-α. Soluble forms of TNFRI and TNFRII naturally exist, such as p75, a monomeric molecule which acts to competitively inhibit the binding of TNF-α and LT-α to cell surface receptors. However, the presence of these inhibitors is not sufficient to block the activity of elevated levels TNF-α [21].

Etanercept prevents TNF-α mediated cellular responses – and modulates the activity of other inflammatory cytokines that are regulated by TNF-α – by competitively binding and neutralizing both free and membrane bound TNF-α, thereby preventing interaction with its cell surface receptors [25, 86]. Although etanercept does bind to both soluble and membrane bound forms of TNF-α, etanercept is believed to primarily bind to the soluble version [43]. Through its effects on TNF-α, etanercept suppresses the expression of molecules involved in inflammation such as adhesion molecules responsible for leukocyte migration such as E-selectin and intercellular adhesion molecule-1 (ICAM-1), serum levels of cytokines (IL-6), and serum levels of matrix metalloproteinase-3 (MMP-3) [33]. Despite the presence of an Fc region, a component of

IgG1 that can induce complement, etanercept does not promote complement mediated cell lysis *in vitro* [33, 87].

The dimeric structure of etanercept allows binding of two molecules of TNF-α at an affinity of 50–1,000 times greater than p75 accounting for the greater inhibitory activity of etanercept than the natural soluble receptor [88, 89]. Etanercept also binds to LT-α preventing the interaction of LT-α with its respective receptors, further attenuating the inflammatory response [33]. From a pharmacological standpoint, the ability of etanercept to bind to LT-α highlights a key difference between etanercept and both adalimumab and infliximab.

TNF binding monoclonal antibodies

Monoclonal antibodies exert pharmacological effects by multiple mechanisms that include direct modulation of the target antigen, antibody dependent cellular cytotoxicity (ADCC) and complement dependent cytotoxicity (CDC) [41]. Often, monoclonal antibodies act through multiple collaborative mechanisms and may exhibit cooperativity with concurrent therapies. In addition to neutralizing the effects of TNF-α, both adalimumab and infliximab appear to have CDC and ADCC activity [40].

Adalimumab and TNF-α neutralization

Adalimumab binds to both soluble and membrane bound TNF-α and is believed to exert its pharmacological effects by specifically binding to soluble TNF-α, thereby preventing its interaction with TNFR1 and TNFR2 [36]. By inhibiting the binding of TNF-α to TNFR1 and TNFR2, the inflammatory response is attenuated resulting in a decrease in inflammatory acute phase reactants such as C-reactive protein, erythrocyte sedimentation rate and interlukin-6 [36]. Furthermore, administration of adalimumab results in a 50% decrease in serum levels of matrix metalloproteinases, mediators of inflammation also involved in joint destruction in patients with RA [90].

Infliximab and TNF-α neutralization

Infliximab binds to both soluble and membrane bound forms of TNF-α preventing the interaction of TNF-α with TNFR1 or TNFR2. The bond formed between infliximab and TNF-α is sustained, reducing the likelihood of dissociation and subsequent activity of bioactive TNF-α. Therefore, the production of inflammatory cytokines that follows TNF-α-TNFR binding, is likely diminished [26].

In addition to binding to trimeric forms of TNF-α, infliximab is also believed to bind to monomeric forms of soluble and membrane bound TNF-α [43]. By binding to TNF-α monomers infliximab may slow or even prevent association of monomeric subunits to form bioactive trimeric TNF-α [43]. As a result, infliximab's therapeutic efficacy may be potentially enhanced.

In patients with RA and Crohn's disease, treatment with infliximab causes a decrease in white blood cell migration, NFκB activity, bone marrow CD3 production and bowel or synovial infiltrates [91, 92]. Furthermore, decreased expression of E-selectin, ICAM-1, MMP-3, and molecules involved in chemoattraction [IL-8 and monocyte chemotactic protein-1 (MCP-1)] were found in patients with Crohn's disease and RA after treatment with infliximab [38].

CDC and ADCC of adalimumab and infliximab

The Fc component of monoclonal antibodies appears to mediate the effector functions of ADCC and CDC. ADCC is induced by cross-linking the Fc gamma receptor on immune effector cells with monoclonal antibody cells. CDC is initiated by binding of the complement protein, C1q, to the monoclonal Fc domain. In particular, monoclonal antibodies of IgG1 isotype are known to have high CDC activity [93]. Binding assays have revealed that both adalimumab and infliximab bind to Fc receptors and C1q in the presence of TNF [40], a property that etanercept does not have. Therefore, as a result of the stable binding of Fc receptors and C1q by monoclonal antibodies, it is believed that adalimumab and infliximab induce ADCC and CDC of TNF producing cells [40].

Effector function is thought to be of critical importance to the success of monoclonal antibodies in certain applications. Unlike etanercept, infliximab induces apoptosis of activated T lymphocytes and cell cycle arrest in a human T cell line [94]. The ability of infliximab to bind to membrane bound TNF-α appears to affect apoptosis as dose-dependent increases in apoptosis and caspase-3 activity, a proteolytic enzyme, were found in monocytes from patients with Crohn's disease following infliximab administration [95]. Although both etanercept and infliximab are potent inhibitors of soluble TNF-α, only infliximab has demonstrated efficacy in Crohn's disease. Therefore, the superior level of effectiveness of infliximab in patients with Crohn's disease has been partly attributed to effector function [96, 97].

Conclusion

The TNF-α antagonists have proven to be a powerful therapeutic advance in treating inflammatory diseases. Advances gained from studying the effects and activities of TNF-α antagonists have provided insights into the pathogenesis of inflammatory diseases. Significant strides have also been made in the realm of TNF-α antagonist pharmacokinetics and have been summarized in Table 2. Continued research into the pharmacokinetics of these therapeutic proteins may act to enhance the understanding of efficacy, tolerability and safety of therapeutic proteins. Further advancements in structural and pharmacological understanding of TNF-α antagonists may also facilitate a greater understanding of inflammatory disease pathogenesis and may one day, lead to a cure for these debilitating disorders.

Table 2. Summary of the Pharmacological Properties of adalimumab, etanercept and infliximab

Variable	Adalimumab	Etanercept	Infliximab
Composition	Human monoclonal IgG1 to TNF [36]	Fusion protein consisting of two soluble domains of the human p75 TNF-receptor linked to the Fc portion of IgG1 [33]	Chimeric monoclonal IgG1 to TNF [38]
Molecular weight (kDa)	148 [36]	150 [33]	149 [38]
Binding specificity	Soluble and membrane bound TNF [35]	Soluble and membrane bound TNF, LT [11]	Soluble and membrane bound TNF [26]
Binding, K_D(M)	7.05×10^{-11} [42]	[A]I. 1.15×10^{-9} [43] [B]II. 2.35×10^{-11} [44]	I. 4.5×10^{-10} [43] II. 1.17×10^{-10} [44]
Peak serum concentration (mcg/mL)	[C]7.7 ± 3.4 at 90 ± 48 h [63]	[D]4.90 ± 2.5 at 69 ± 48 h [54]	[E]165 ± 42 [57]
Average serum concentration (mcg/mL)	[C]5.5 ± 2.5 [63]	[D]3.67 ± 0.7 [54]	[F]27.0 [57]
Minimum serum concentration (mcg/mL)	[C]3.8 ± 2.1 [63]	3.10 ± 1.6 [54]	[G]8.3 ± 11.9 [57]
Immunogenicity (Antibody formation percentage)	6–12% [49]	0–2% [49, 50]	8–68% [53]
Administration	SC injection [36]	SC injection [33]	IV infusion [38]
Bioavailability (%)	64 [36]	58 [68]	–
Apparent volume of distribution (L)	4.7–6.0 [36]	12 ± 6 [75]	3.0–5.0 [38]
Half-Life (days)	14.0 [36]	4.25 ± 1.25 [33	8.0–9.5 [38]
Mechanism of action	A. Binding and neutralizing soluble TNF alpha [36] B. ADCC and CDC mediated lysis of TNF [40]	A. Binding and neutralizing both free and membrane bound TNF, and LT [33]	A. Binding and neutralizing soluble and membrane bound TNF-α [98] B. Induces apoptosis of monocytes [99] and T-cells in Crohn's disease [94], decreasing the formation of TNF-α C. ADCC and CDC mediated lysis of TNF [40]

(Continued on next page)

Table 2. (Continued)

Variable	Adalimumab	Etanercept	Infliximab
Elimination	Follows course of other IgG molecules [36]	Metabolized through a peptide and amino acid pathway with either recycling of amino acids or elimination in bile and urine [75]	Follows course of other IgG molecules
Elimination rate (mL/h)	12 [36]	160 ± 80 [33]	–

Note: SC = subcutaneous; IV = intravenous; h = hours
[A, B] Controversy exists in the literature as to whether etanercept or infliximab has a greater K_D [43, 44]. Conflicting values are presented.
[C] RA patients, steady state, 40 mg every other week. Psoriasis information unavailable at the time of publication. Psoriasis patients may metabolize the drug differently from RA patients.
[D] Psoriasis patients, steady state, 50 mg biweekly
[E] Psoriasis patients, 5 mg/kg post 2nd infusion
[F] Psoriasis patients, during the first 26 weeks, with 5 mg/kg doses at weeks 0, 2 & 6
[G] Psoriasis patients, at week 14, following 5 mg/kg doses at weeks 0, 2 & 6

Acknowledgements
The authors wish to thank Dr. Neil Shear and Dr. Jeffrey Weinberg for their critical review of the manuscript.

References

1 Ware CF (2003) The TNF superfamily. *Cytokine Growth Factor Rev* 14(3–4): 181–184
2 Abbas AK, Lichtman AH (2003) *Cellular and molecular immunology*. Saunders, Philadelphia
3 Vassalli P (1992) The pathophysiology of tumor necrosis factor. *Annu Rev Immunol* 10: 411–452
4 Paul NL, Ruddle NH (1988) Lymphotoxin. *Annu Rev Immunol* 6: 407–438
5 Smith CA, Farrah T, Goodwin RG (1994) The TNF receptor superfamily of cellular and viral proteins: activation, costimulation, and death. *Cell* 76: 959
6 Ware CF, Crowe PD, Grayson MH, Androlewicz MJ, Browning JL (1992) Expression of surface lymphotoxin and tumor necrosis factor on activated T, B, and natural killer cells. *J Immunol* 149: 3881–3888
7 Browning JL, Ngam-ek A, Lawton P, DeMarinis J, Tizard R, Chow EP, Hession C, O'Brine-Greco B, Foley SF, Ware CF (1993) Lymphotoxin b, a novel member of the TNF family that forms a heteromeric complex with lymphotoxin on the cell surface. *Cell* 72: 847–856
8 Ito D, Back TC, Shakhov AN, Wiltrout RH, Nedospasov SA (1999) Mice with a targeted mutation in lymphotoxin-alpha exhibit enhanced tumor growth and metastasis: impaired NK cell development and recruitment. *J Immunol* 1: 163(5): 2809–2815
9 Vandenabeele P, Declercq W, Beyaert R, Fiers W (1995) Two tumour necrosis factor receptors: structure and function. *Trends Cell Biol* 5(10): 392–399
10 Franki AS, Van Beneden K, Dewint P, Meeus I, Veys E, Deforce D, Elewaut D (2005) Lymphotoxin alpha 1 beta 2: a critical mediator in V alpha 14i NKT cell differentiation. *Mol Immunol* 42(4): 413–417
11 Gudbrandsdottir S, Bliddal H, Petri A, Terslev L, Danneskiold-Samsoe B, Bjornhart B, Bendtzen K, Muller K (2004) Plasma TNF binding capacity profiles during treatment with etanercept in rheumatoid arthritis. *Scand J Rheumatol* 33(6): 385–388
12 Gottlieb AB, Chamian F, Masud S, Cardinale I, Abello MV, Lowes MA, Chen F, Magliocco M, Krueger JG (2005) TNF inhibition rapidly down-regulates multiple proinflammatory pathways in psoriasis plaques. *J Immunol* 175(4): 2721–2729
13 Mease P (2002) Psoriatic arthritis: the role of TNF inhibition and the effect of its inhibition with etanercept. *Clin Exp Rheumatol* 20(6 Suppl 28): S116–S121
14 Rutgeerts P, Van Assche G, Vermeire S (2004) Optimizing anti-TNF treatment in inflammatory bowel disease. *Gastroenterology* 126(6): 1593–1610
15 Kawaguchi M, Mitsuhashi Y, Kondo S (2005) Overexpression of tumor necrosis-alpha converting enzyme in psoriasis. *British Journal of Dermatology* 152 (5): 915–919
16 Xu H, Sethi JK, Hotamisligil GS (1999) Transmembrane tumor necrosis factor (TNF)-alpha inhibits adipocyte differentiation by selectively activating TNF receptor 1. *J Biol Chem* 274(37): 26287–26295
17 Shetty A, Forbes A (2002) Pharmacogenomics of response to anti-tumor necrosis factor therapy in patients with Crohn's disease. *Am J Pharmacogenomics* 2(4): 215–221
18 Mease P (2004) TNF-alpha therapy in psoriatic arthritis and psoriasis. *Ann Rheum Dis* 63(7): 755 –758
19 Yamauchi PS, Gindi V, Lowe NJ (2004) The treatment of psoriasis and psoriatic arthritis with etanercept: practical considerations on monotherapy, combination therapy, and safety. *Dermatol Clin* 4: 449–459
20 Aderka D, Engelmann H, Maor Y, Brakebusch C, Wallach D (1992) Stabilization of the bioactivity of tumor necrosis factor by its soluble receptors. *J Exp Med* 1: 175(2): 323–329
21 Baugh JA, Bucala R (2001) Mechanisms for modulating TNF alpha in immune and inflammatory disease. *Curr Opin Drug Discov Devel* 4(5): 635–650
22 Sieper J, Van den Brande J (2005) Diverse effects of infliximab and etanercept on T lymphocytes. *Semin Arthritis Rheum* 34(5 Pt 2): 23–27
23 Ettehadi P, Greaves WM, Wallach D, Aderka D, Camp RDR (1994) Elevated tumor necrosis factor-alpha (TNF-alpha) biological activity in psoriatic skin lesions. *Clin Exp Immunol* 96: 146–151

24 Partsch G, Steiner G, Leeb BF, Dunky F, Broll H, Smolen JS (1997) Highly increased levels of tumor necrosis factor-alpha and other proinflammatory cytokines in psoriatic arthritis synovial fluid. *J Rheumatol* 24(3): 518–523

25 Goffe B, Cather JC (2003) Etanercept: An overview. *J Am Acad Dermatol* 49(2 Suppl): S105–S111

26 Winterfield L, Menter A (2004) Psoriasis and its treatment with infliximab-mediated tumor necrosis factor alpha blockade. *Dermatol Clin* 4: 437–447, ix

27 Mease P (2004) TNF-alpha therapy in psoriatic arthritis and psoriasis. *Ann Rheum Dis* 63(7): 755 –758

28 Dayer JM, Beutler B, Cerami A (1985) Cachectin/tumor necrosis factor stimulates collagenase and prostaglandin E2 production by human synovial cells and dermal fibroblasts. *J Exp Med* 1;162(6); 2163–2168

29 Bertolini DR, Nedwin GE, Bringman TS, Smith DD, Mundy GR (1986) Stimulation of bone resorption and inhibition of bone formation *in vitro* by human tumour necrosis factors. *Nature* 319(6053): 516–518

30 Catrina AI, Lampa J, Ernestam S, af Klint E, Bratt J, Klareskog L, Ulfgren AK (2002) Anti-tumour necrosis factor (TNF)-alpha therapy (etanercept) down-regulates serum matrix metalloproteinase (MMP)-3 and MMP-1 in rheumatoid arthritis. *Rheumatology (Oxford)* 41(5): 484–489

31 Ina K, Itoh J, Fukushima K, Kusugami K, Yamaguchi T, Kyokane K, Imada A, Binion DG, Musso A, West GA et al (1999) Resistance of Crohn's disease T cells to multiple apoptotic signals is associated with a Bcl-2/Bax mucosal imbalance. *J Immunol* 163(2): 1081–1090

32 Soderholm JD, Streutker C, Yang PC, Paterson C, Singh PK, McKay DM, Sherman PM, Croitoru K, Perdue MH (2004) Increased epithelial uptake of protein antigens in the ileum of Crohn's disease mediated by tumour necrosis factor alpha. *Gut* 53(12): 1817–1824

33 ENBREL® (etanercept). Product monograph. Amgen Inc., Thousand Oaks, CA, July, 2003

34 Rau R (2002) Adalimumab (a fully human anti-tumor necrosis factor alpha monoclonal antibody) in the treatment of active rheumatoid arthritis: the initial results of five trials. *Ann Rheum Dis* 61(Suppl 2): ii70–ii73

35 Sandborn WJ (2005) New concepts in anti-tumor necrosis factor therapy for inflammatory bowel disease. *Rev Gastroenterol Disord* 5(1): 10–18

36 HUMIRA® (adalimumab) product monograph. Abbott Laboratories, North Chicago, IL, February 2005

37 Gottlieb AB (2003) Infliximab for psoriasis. *J Am Acad Dermatol* 49(2 Suppl): S112–S117

38 REMICAIDE® (infliximab) product monograph. Centocor, Inc., Malvern, PA 19355, USA, 2001

39 Santora LC, Kaymakcalan Z, Sakorafas P, Krull IS, Grant K (2001) Characterization of noncovalent complexes of recombinant human monoclonal antibody and antigen using cation exchange, size exclusion chromatography, and BIAcore. *Anal Biochem* 299(2): 119–129

40 Kohno T, Stevens SR, Louie JS (2005) Adalimumab and infliximab bind to Fc-receptor and C1q and generate immunoprecipitation–A different mechanism from etanercept [abstract]. *J Am Acad Dermatol* 52(3): 400

41 Roskos LK, Davis GC, Schwab GM (2004) The clinical pharmacology of therapeutic monoclonal antibodies. *Drug Development Research* 61: 108–120

42 Granneman RG, Zhang Y, Noertersheuser PA, Velagapudi RB, Awni WM, Locke CS (2003) Pharmacokinetic/pharmacodynamic (PK/PD) relationships of adalimumab (Humira™) in rheumatoid arthritis (RA) patients during II/III clinical trials [abstract]. *Arthritis Rheum* 48 Suppl: S140

43 Scallon B, Cai A, Solowski N, Rosenberg A, Song XY, Shealy D, Wagner C (2002) Binding and functional comparisons of two types of tumor necrosis factor antagonists. *J Pharmacol Exp Ther* 301(2): 418–426

44 Smith TD, Friend D, Smith CA (2002) Comparative TNF Binding Characteristics of Etanercept (Enbrel) and Infliximab (Remicade). *European Congress of Rheumatology*. Abstract 98101 [EULAR]

45 Schellekens H (2002) Immunogenicity of therapeutic proteins: clinical implications and future prospects. *Clin Ther* 24(11): 1720–1740; discussion 1719

46 Porter S (2001) Human immune response to recombinant human proteins. *J Pharm Sci* 90: 1–11

47 Dillman RO (1990) Human antimouse and antiglobulin response to monoclonal antibodies. *Antibody Immunocon Radiopharm* 3: 1–15

48 Weiner LM (1999) Monoclonal antibody therapy of cancer. *Semin Oncol* 26(5 Suppl 14): 43–51

49 Anderson PJ (2005) Tumor necrosis factor inhibitors: Clinical implications of their different immunogenicity profiles. *Semin Arthritis Rheum* 34(5 Pt 2): 19–22
50 Foerder C, Rogge M (2002) Immunogenicity of Enbrel: clinical trial observations. *Annual European Congress of Rheumatology*, 2002 [EULAR]
51 Sorbera LA, Rabasseda X, Castaner RM (2001) Adalimumab: antiarthritic treatment of IBD. *Drugs Future* 26(7): 639–646
52 Anderson PJ (2005) Tumor necrosis factor inhibitors: Clinical implications of their different immunogenicity profiles. *Semin Arthritis Rheum* 34(5 Pt 2): 19–22
53 Farrell RJ, Alsahli M, Jeen YT, Falchuk KR, Peppercorn MA, Michetti P (2003) Intravenous hydrocortisone premedication reduces antibodies to infliximab in Crohn's disease: a randomized controlled trial. *Gastroenterology* 124(4): 917–924
54 Nestorov I (2005) Clinical pharmacokinetics of tumor necrosis factor antagonists. *J Rheumatol* Suppl 74: 13–18
55 Lobo ED, Hansen RJ, Balthasar JP (2004) Antibody pharmacokinetics and pharmacodynamics. *J Pharm Sci* 93(11): 2645–2668
56 Nestorov I (2005) Clinical pharmacokinetics of TNF antagonists: How do they differ? *Semin Arthritis Rheum* 34(5 Pt 2): 12–18
57 DiNoto D, Mace K, DeRita R, Jordan R, Wagner C (1999) Pharmacokinetics of infliximab, a chimeric monoclonal antibody specific to tumor necrosis factor: clinical studies in rheumatoid arthritis patients. *AAPS Annual Meeting*; November 1999. Abstract 4733. [APPS PharmSci]
58 Kavanaugh A, St Clair EW, McCune WJ, Braakman T, Lipsky P (2000) Chimeric anti-tumor necrosis factor-alpha monoclonal antibody treatment of patients with rheumatoid arthritis receiving methotrexate therapy. *J Rheumatol* 27(4): 841–850
59 Schwab M, Klotz U (2001) Pharmacokinetic considerations in the treatment of inflammatory bowel disease. *Clin Pharmacokinet* 40(19): 723–751
60 Fasanmade AA, Zhu YW, Wagner C, Pendley C, Davis HM (2002) Population pharmacokinetics of single dose infliximab in patients with Crohn's disease. ASCPT 2002 abstracts, abstract TPII-92. *Clin Pharmacol Ther* 71: P66
61 Porter CJ, Charman SA (2000) Lymphatic transport of proteins after subcutaneous administration. *J Pharm Sci* 89(3): 297–310
62 Supersaxo A, Hein WR, Steffen H (1990) Effect of molecular weight on the lymphatic absorption of water-soluble compounds following subcutaneous administration. *Pharm Res* 7(2): 167–169
63 Velgapudi RB, Noertersheuser PA, Awni WM, Kupper H, Granneman GR, van de Putte LB (2003) The effect of methotrexate (MTX) coadministration on the pharmacokinetics (PK) of adalimumab (HUMIRA) following a single intravenous injection to rheumatoid arthritis patients. *ACR Annual Scientific Meeting*; November 2003, Orlando, FL. Poster 258
64 Lobo ED, Hansen RJ, Balthasar JP (2004) Antibody pharmacokinetics and pharmacodynamics. *J Pharm Sci* 93(11): 2645–2668
65 Lin YS, Nguyen C, Mendoza JL, Escandon E, Fei D, Meng YG, Modi NB (1999) Preclinical pharmacokinetics, interspecies scaling, and tissue distribution of a humanized monoclonal antibody against vascular endothelial growth factor. *J Pharmacol Exp Ther* 1: 371–378
66 Pepin S, Lutsch C, Grandgeorge M, Scherrmann JM (1995) Snake F(ab')2 antivenom from hyperimmunized horse: pharmacokinetics following intravenous and intramuscular administrations in rabbits. *Pharm Res* 10: 1470–1473
67 Vaishnaw AK, TenHoor CN (2002) Pharmacokinetics, biologic activity, and tolerability of alefacept by intravenous and intramuscular administration. *J Pharmacokinet Pharmacodyn* 29(5–6): 415–426
68 Lebsack ME, Hanna RK, Lange MA, Newman A, Ji W, Korth-Bradley JM (1997) Absolute bioavailability of TNF receptor fusion protein following subcutaneous injection in healthy volunteers [abstract 233]. *Pharmacotherapy* 17: 1118
69 Fasano A (1998) Novel approaches for oral delivery of macromolecules. *J Pharm Sci* 87(11): 1351 –1356
70 Mahato RI, Narang AS, Thoma L, Miller DD (2003) Emerging trends in oral delivery of peptide and protein drugs. *Crit Rev Ther Drug Carrier Syst* 20(2–3): 153–214
71 McMartin C (1992) Pharmacokinetics of peptides and proteins: Opportunities and challenges. *Adv Drug Res* 22: 39–106
72 Tang L, Persky AM, Hochhaus G, Meibohm B (2004) Pharmacokinetic aspects of biotechnology products. *J Pharm Sci* 93(9): 2184–2204

73 Zito SW (1997) *Pharmaceutical biotechnology: A programmed text.* Technomic Pub Co, Lancaster, PA
74 Reilly RM, Sandhu J, Alvarez-Diez TM, Gallinger S, Kirsh J, Stern H (1995) Problems of delivery of monoclonal antibodies. Pharmaceutical and pharmacokinetic solutions. *Clin Pharmacokinet* 28(2): 126–142
75 Korth-Bradley JM, Rubin AS, Hanna RK, Simcoe DK, Lebsack ME (2000) The pharmacokinetics of etanercept in healthy volunteers. *Ann Pharmacother* 34(2): 161–164
76 Rowland M, Tozer TN (eds) (1995) *Clinical Pharmacokinetics: Concepts and Applications*, 3rd ed. Lippincott Williams & Wilkins, Philadelphia
77 LaDuca JR, Gaspari AA (2001) Targeting tumor necrosis factor alpha. New drugs used to modulate inflammatory diseases. *Dermatol Clin* 19(4): 617–635
78 Waldmann TA, Strober W (1969) Metabolism of immunoglobulins. *Prog Allergy* 13: 1–110
79 Wagner CL, Schantz A, Barnathan E, Olson A, Mascelli MA, Ford J, Damaraju L, Schaible T, Maini RN, Tcheng JE (2003) Consequences of immunogenicity to the therapeutic monoclonal antibodies ReoPro and Remicade. *Dev Biol* (Basel) 112: 37–53
80 Saripalli YV, Gaspari AA (2005) Focus on: biologics that affect therapeutic agents in dermatology. *J Drugs Dermatol* 4(2): 233–245
81 Zhu X, Meng G, Dickinson BL, Li X, Mizoguchi E, Miao L, Wang Y, Robert C, Wu B, Smith PD et al (2001) MHC class I-related neonatal Fc receptor for IgG is functionally expressed in monocytes, intestinal macrophages, and dendritic cells. *J Immunol* 166(5): 3266–3276
82 Junghans RP (1997) Finally! The Brambell receptor (FcRB). Mediator of transmission of immunity and protection from catabolism for IgG. *Immunol Res* 16(1): 29–57
83 Ward ES, Zhou J, Ghetie V, Ober RJ (2003) Evidence to support the cellular mechanism involved in serum IgG homeostasis in humans. *Int Immunol* 15(2): 187–195
84 Smith RA, Baglioni C (1987) The active form of tumor necrosis factor is a trimer. *J Biol Chem* 262: 6951–6954
85 Pennica D, Kohr WJ, Fendly BM, Shire SJ, Raab HE, Borchardt PE, Lewis M, Goeddel DV (1992) Characterization of a recombinant extracellular domain of the type 1 tumor necrosis factor receptor: evidence for tumor necrosis factor-alpha induced receptor aggregation. *Biochemistry* 31: 1134–1141
86 Papp KA (2004) Etanercept in psoriasis. *Expert Opin Pharmacother* 5(10): 2139–2146
87 Scallon BJ, Moore MA, Trinh H, Knight DM, Ghrayeb J (1995) Chimeric anti-TNF-alpha monoclonal antibody cA2 binds recombinant transmembrane TNF-alpha and activates immune effector functions. *Cytokine* 7: 251–259
88 Mohler KM, Torrance DS, Smith CA, Goodwin RG, Stremler KE, Fung VP, Madani H, Widmer MB (1993) Soluble tumor necrosis factor (TNF) receptors are effective therapeutic agents in lethal endotoxemia and function simultaneously as both TNF carriers and TNF antagonists. *J Immunol* 151(3): 1548–1561
89 Peppel K, Crawford D, Beutler B (1991) A tumor necrosis factor (TNF) receptor-IgG heavy chain chimeric protein as a bivalent antagonist of TNF activity. *J Exp Med* 174(6): 1483–1489
90 Kempeni J (2000) Update on D2E7: a fully human anti-tumour necrosis factor alpha monoclonal antibody. *Ann Rheum Dis* 59 (Suppl I): i44–i45
91 Jacobsen FW, Rothe M, Rusten L, Goeddel DV, Smeland EB, Veiby OP, Slordal L, Jacobsen SE (1994) Role of the 75-kDa tumor necrosis factor receptor: inhibition of early hematopoiesis. *Proc Natl Acad Sci USA* 91(22): 10695–10699
92 Newland MR, Weinstein A, Kerdel F (2002) Rapid response to infliximab in severe pustular psoriasis, von Zumbusch type. *Int J Dermatol* 41: 449–452
93 Presta LG (2002) Engineering antibodies for therapy. *Curr Pharm Biotechnol* 3(3): 237–256
94 Van den Brande JM, Braat H, van den Brink GR, Versteeg HH, Bauer CA, Hoedemaeker I, van Montfrans C, Hommes DW, Peppelenbosch MP, van Deventer SJ (2003) Infliximab but not etanercept induces apoptosis in lamina propria T-lymphocytes from patients with Crohn's disease. *Gastroenterology* 124(7): 1774–1785
95 Lügering A, Schmidt M, Lügering N, Pauels HG, Domschke W, Kucharzik T (2001) Infliximab induces apoptosis in monocytes from patients with chronic active Crohn's disease by using a caspase-dependent pathway. *Gastroenterology* 121: 1145–1157
96 Sandborn WJ, Hanauer SB, Katz S, Safdi M, Wolf DG, Baerg RD, Tremaine WJ, Johnson T, Diehl NN, Zinsmeister AR (2001) Etanercept for active Crohn's disease: a randomized, double-blind, placebo-controlled trial. *Gastroenterology* 21(5): 1088–1094
97 Su CG, Judge TA, Lichtenstein GR (2001) The role of biological therapy in inflammatory bowel

disease. *Drugs Today (Barc)* 37(2): 121–133
98 Maini RN, Feldmann M (2002) How does infliximab work in rheumatoid arthritis? *Arthritis Res.* 4 Suppl 2: S22–S28
99 Shen C, Assche GV, Colpaert S, Maerten P, Geboes K, Rutgeerts P, Ceuppens JL (2005) Adalimumab induces apoptosis of human monocytes: a comparative study with infliximab and etanercept. *Aliment Pharmacol Ther* 21(3): 251–258

TNF-alpha Inhibitors
Edited by Jeffrey M. Weinberg and Robin Buchholz

Etanercept in rheumatology

Jeffrey D. Greenberg and Mitsumasa Kishimoto

NYU Hospital for Joint Diseases, New York, USA

Introduction

Etanercept has been studied in a broad range of rheumatologic conditions since its development. Etanercept was first approved by the United States Food and Drug Administration (FDA) in 1998 for the treatment of active adult rheumatoid arthritis (RA), and was subsequently approved by the European Medicines Evaluation Agency (EMEA). Since its initial approval for adult RA, etanercept has also been approved by the FDA and EMEA for three other indications including polyarticular juvenile idiopathic arthritis, psoriatic arthritis and ankylosing spondylitis. Etanercept has also been studied in other rheumatic diseases, but has not yet been approved for these indications. This chapter will address the four rheumatologic conditions for which etanercept has been approved by regulatory authorities.

Rationale for etanercept in rheumatic diseases

Administration of TNF-α antagonists including etanercept for immune-mediated rheumatic conditions including RA, psoriatic arthritis (PsA), juvenile idiopathic arthritis (JIA) and ankylosing spondylitis (AS) represent rational, mechanism-based therapies.

Although the role of TNF-α has been most extensively studied in RA, the pivotal role of TNF-α in regulating 'downstream' inflammatory mediators has recently been confirmed for other diseases as well. Predominantly studied in synovial cultures, TNF-α antagonism has been shown to reduce 'downstream' cytokines and other mediators including interleukin-6, interleukin-1, interleukin-8, monocyte chemoattractant protein-1, and vascular endothelial growth factor [1]. Similar to the presence of TNF-α in the synovial fluid from RA patients, TNF-α is also highly expressed in the synovial fluid of PsA patients [2]. In contrast to RA and PsA, studies of serum and synovial levels of TNF-α and other proinflammatory cytokines have reported conflicting results, particularly with respect to serum levels of TNF-α [3]. In JIA, there is evidence of abundant TNF-α expression within synovial tissue and a high level of the p55 TNF receptor on the synovial endothelial cells [4]. While the detailed mechanisms of action have not been fully elucidated and may vary across rheumatic diseases, randomized clinical trials have clearly defined a role for TNF-α antagonism in RA, PsA, JIA and AS.

Rheumatoid arthritis

Epidemiology and clinical features

Rheumatoid arthritis (RA) is an autoimmune disease of unknown etiology characterized by chronic inflammation of the synovial lining of the joints and destruction of the cartilage and bone. RA affects approximately 1% of the adult population [5]. The disease course is generally chronic with fluctuations in severity, resulting in progressive pain and disability in the majority of patients. The pattern of joint involvement in RA is typically symmetric involving small joints, frequently resulting in clinical deformities. Numerous studies have observed that the life expectancy in RA patients is diminished. The most frequent cause of death in RA patients are cardiovascular-related causes [6, 7]. In addition to the associated risk of cardiovascular disease, RA has also been linked to an increased risk of lymphoma in multiple studies [8, 9].

Clinical trials of etanercept monotherapy

The efficacy of etanercept monotherapy and etanercept combination therapy with methotrexate has been demonstrated in multiple randomized clinical trials (RCTs). The first multicenter, placebo-controlled RCT of etanercept was a Phase II trial involving randomization to one of three etanercept doses (0.25 mg/m^2, 2 mg/m^2 or 16 mg/m^2) *versus* placebo [10]. Among patients receiving the 16 mg/m^2 dose of etanercept, 75% achieved an American College of Rheumatology (ACR) 20% improvement, which was superior to rates for the lower doses and placebo. The definition of the ACR 20% improvement is summarized in Figure 1. Subsequently, a Phase III trial was conducted, randomizing RA patients to etanercept 10 mg or 25 mg subcutaneously twice weekly *versus* placebo [11]. Entry criteria included an inadequate response to one of four disease-modifying anti-rheumatic drugs (DMARDs) with a 1 month DMARD washout, as well as high disease activity, defined by minimum joint counts and other measures. ACR 20 response rates at 6 months were 59% for etanercept 25 mg, 51% for etanercept 10 mg and 11% for placebo ($p < 0.001$ for both etanercept arms *versus* placebo). For etanercept 25 mg, the ACR 50 and 70 response rates were 40% and 15%, respectively.

The Early Rheumatoid Arthritis (ERA) trial compared etanercept monotherapy to methotrexate monotherapy for patients with less than 3 years duration of RA [12]. The primary study results were reported at 12 months by Bathon et al. Patients (n = 632) were randomized to etanercept 10 mg, etanercept

Requires ≥20% improvement of:

- **Swollen joint count**
- **Tender joint count**
- **≥20% improvement in 3 of the following 5 criteria:**
  - **Patient global assessment of disease activity**
  - **Physician global assessment of disease activity**
  - **Patient assessment of pain**
  - **Acute phase reactant (ESR or CRP)**
  - **Patient assessment of disability (HAQ)**

Figure 1. The American College of Rheumatology Definition of Improvement* in Rheumatoid Arthritis. * This is the definition for an ACR 20% improvement. Similar calculations are made for ACR 50% and ACR 70% improvements. Abbreviations: ESR = erythrocyte sedimentation rate; CRP = C-reactive protein; HAQ = Health Assessment Questionnaire. Source: Felson DT et al. (1995) *Arthritis Rheum* 38: 727–735

25 mg or methotrexate 7.5 mg weekly, which was rapidly escalated to 20 mg by week 8. At 12 months, the ACR 20% response favored etanercept 25 mg (72%) *versus* methotrexate (65%), but was not statistically significant ($p = 0.16$). In contrast, superior efficacy was evident after 2 years, achieved by 72% on etanercept 25 mg *versus* 59% on methotrexate ($p = 0.005$) In addition, differences in radiographic outcomes were noted. After 24 months, the mean change from baseline in total Sharp scores was 1.3 units for etanercept 25 mg *versus* 3.2 units for methotrexate ($p = 0.001$).

Clinical trials of etanercept combination therapy with methotrexate

Subsequent clinical trials of etanercept in RA patients were conducted in combination with methotrexate. The first study to demonstrate superior efficacy of etanercept plus methotrexate compared to methotrexate alone was a 24-week, double-blind RCT of 89 patients [13]. All patients were required to be taking stable doses of methotrexate between 15–25 mg weekly. ACR 20% response rates were 71% for etanercept plus methotrexate *versus* 27% for methotrexate alone ($P < 0.001$). ACR 50% and 70% responses were achieved by 39% and 15% of patients in the etanercept/methotrexate arm *versus* 3% and 0% of patients in the methotrexate alone arm ($p < 0.05$ for both). The Trial of Etanercept and Methotrexate with Radiographic Patient Outcomes (TEMPO) further examined the efficacy of etanercept *versus* methotrexate *versus* combination therapy. This multi-centered, double blind trial included 682 patients [14]. At 12 months, ACR 20% response rates were highest for the combination of etanercept and methotrexate (85%) *versus* etanercept monotherapy (76%) *versus* methotrexate monotherapy (75%). For patients on etanercept and methotrexate, ACR 50% and 70% response rates were 69% and 43%, respectively. A total of 35% of patients on this combination achieved criteria for RA clinical remission. Similarly, radiographic outcomes, defined by the mean change in total Sharp score, were superior for the combination therapy arm (–0.5) *versus* etanercept (0.5) *versus* methotrexate (2.8). Based on the results of TEMPO, combination therapy of methotrexate with etanercept appears to maximize efficacy outcomes in RA.

Psoriatic arthritis

Epidemiology and clinical features

Psoriatic arthritis (PsA) is a chronic inflammatory arthritis associated with psoriasis, frequently characterized by bony proliferation and osteolysis at tendon, ligament and capsule inertions (entheses). The inflammatory arthritis can present in a variety of patterns including large joint oligoarticular arthritis, small-joint polyarticular arthritis (rheumatoid-like), distal interphalangeal arthritis, sacroiliitis, spondylitis and arthritis mutilans, frequently accompanied by dactylitis and enthesitis [15]. Studies of the prevalence of arthritis among patients with pre-existing psoriasis have observed prevalence rates ranging from 5–42%, likely due to non-uniformity of case definition. In addition, observations of the severity of the arthritis have been conflicting, particularly with respect to the development of erosive arthritis. Despite the conflicting data, there is increasing awareness that a subset of PsA patients develop radiographic erosions and clinical deformities that require aggressive, structure-modifying treatment.

Clinical trials of etanercept

Two pivotal randomized, placebo-controlled clinical trials of etanercept in psoriatic arthritis led to the regulatory approval of etanercept for the treatment of PsA [16, 17]. The first trial was a phase II trial of 60 patients, with patients randomized to either placebo or etanercept 25 mg BIW for 12 weeks [16]. Inclusion criteria required at least three swollen or tender joints with inadequate response to non-steroidal anti-inflammatory agents (NSAIDs). Patients were permitted to continue stable doses of methotrexate (= 25 mg per week) or corticosteroids (= 10 mg prednisone per day). The primary outcome for this trial was a 75% improvement in the Psoriatic Arthritis Response Criteria (PsARC) score. The PsARC endpoint is comprised of four measures: 1) patient global assessment, 2) physician global assessment, 3) joint pain/tenderness score and 4) joint swelling score. Achievement of the PsARC endpoint requires improvement in at least two of the four measures, one of which must be joint pain/tenderness or swelling, and no worsening in any of the four measures.

Among patients receiving etanercept, 87% achieved the required 75% PsARC response compared to 13% of placebo-treated patients ($p < 0.001$).

Using the ACR 20% response criteria (see RA section) as a predefined secondary outcome, 73% of patients on etanercept achieved an ACR 20% improvement at 12 weeks *versus* 13% of the placebo group ($p < 0.001$). In addition, skin improvement was evaluated, using a 75% improvement in the Psoriatic Area and Severity Index (PASI) response. A total of 26% of patients receiving etanercept achieved a PASI 75 response, whereas 0% of placebo patients achieved a PASI 75 response ($p = 0.015$).

The second pivotal trial of etanercept in PsA was a larger multi-center, placebo controlled Phase III trial. Inclusion criteria were generally similar to the Phase II trial, but also required a qualifying cutaneous lesion = 2 cm in diameter. A total of 205 patients were randomized to etanercept 25 mg BIW *versus* placebo. This trial included an initial 24-week double blind phase, with a 48-week open-label extension ($n = 168$) for which all patients were eligible. In this study, an ACR 20% improvement was the primary endpoint for the arthritis evaluation. A total of 59% of etanercept-treated patients achieved an ACR-20% response *versus* 15% of placebo-treated patients ($p < 0.001$). Similarly, higher levels of PsARC responses were achieved at 12 and 24 weeks.

In addition to assessment of signs and symptoms, the trial also evaluated radiographic progression using the modified Total Sharp Score (TSS), a radiographic outcome that incorporates both radiographic erosions and joint space narrowing. Whereas the placebo-treated group experienced radiographic progression (mean TSS +1.00 units), the etanercept-treated group did not have radiographic progression at 12 months (mean TSS = –0.03 units, $p < 0.001$). Similar to the Phase II trial, the mean percentage change in PASI score was significantly improved with etanercept (42%) compared to placebo (worsened by 8%, $p < 0.001$). Based on these two pivotal trials, etanercept has been approved by regulatory authorities to reduce the signs and symptoms of active PsA, as well as to inhibit the progression of structural damage associated with PsA.

Juvenile idiopathic arthritis

Epidemiology and clinical features

Juvenile idiopathic arthritis (JIA), formerly known as juvenile rheumatoid arthritis (JRA) or juvenile chronic arthritis, is most common rheumatic disease in children [18, 19]. JIA may be associated with severe disability and life-threatening complications, particularly in patients in whom polyarthritis develops and who do not respond satisfactorily to treatment [20]. The incidence of JIA ranges from 1–22 per 100,000 with prevalence of 8–150 per 100,000 [21–23]. It is characterized by early-onset arthritis (defined as swelling or limitation of motion of joint accompanied by heat, pain, or tenderness before age 16 years) for at least 6 weeks' duration with other identifiable causes of arthritis excluded [24]. The latest classification of the International League of

Association for Rheumatology (ILAR) distinguished seven groups of JIA according to the following: 1) the onset pattern (systemic, and oligoarticular or polyarticular with no systemic symptoms); 2) the presence or absence of rheumatoid factor in polyarticular JIA; 3) a personal or family history of psoriasis, which defines psoriatic JIA; and 4) the presence of enthesitis, sacroiliitis, HLA-B27, or other features that define enthesitis related JIA.

Clinical trials of etanercept

The US FDA approved etanercept for the treatment of moderately to severely active polyarticular-course JIA in patients with inadequate response to one or more disease modifying medicines in 1999. The pivotal study that led to this approval was published in 2000 [25]. In this multicenter, placebo controlled trial, eligible patients were between the ages of 4–17 and had active, polyarticular course JIA. All patients received etanercept 0.4 mg/kg subcutaneously twice weekly for up to 3 months. Patients who met the JIA definition of improvement criteria at the end of 3 months were then randomized to continue on etanercept at the same dose and schedule or to receive placebo until disease flare occurred, or until 4 months elapsed, whichever was earlier. 69 patients enrolled in the trial, and 51 (74%) met the criteria for improvement at 3 months and entered the blinded portion of the trial. A significantly greater number of patients who received placebo had disease flare than did patients who received etanercept. After 2 years of follow-up, patients in the initial trial continue to have an excellent response [26]. In these studies, etanercept treatment was effective regardless of the JIA onset type. On the other hand, an open-label, prospective, multicenter study from France showed that the higher rate of treatment failure in the group with systemic-onset JIA was observed compared to those with oligoarticular or polyarticular onset JIA [27]. Further studies are needed to clarify whether efficacy varies by subtype.

Ankylosing spondylitis

Epidemiology and clinical features

Ankylosing spondylitis (AS), the prototype of the spondyloarthritides (SpA), is a chronic inflammatory disease. It characteristically affects young adults with a peak age of onset between 20–30 years. In the past, the prevalence of SpA may have been under-reported [28]; more recently, the prevalence of the group of SpA as a whole has been calculated to be 0.5–1.9% [29], similar to that of rheumatoid arthritis. The prevalence of AS is most clearly described in the Caucasian ranging from 0.1–1.1% [30]. It depends upon the ethnic group, the prevalence of HLA-B27, the selection of subjects for evaluation, and the criteria for diagnosis [29, 31, 32]. For example, one report found the prevalence of AS in a Northern Norway community in which HLA-B27 was present in 15.9% of individuals [29].

AS is characterized by insidious onset of axial skeletal ankylosis (sacroiliitis), inflammation at the insertions of tendons (enthesitis), and occasionally, peripheral arthritis. AS severity varies with perhaps 30% of patients with severe disease. Like RA, AS causes significant disability in a substantial proportion of patients [33].

In contrast to RA, there are only a few studies on treatment with non-biological DMARDs in AS. Sulfasalazine has limited efficacy in patients with peripheral arthritis and possibly in early disease stages [34]. No studies have provided convincing evidence of the efficacy of methotrexate in AS, although a small open-labeled study suggested that it can be effective in some patients with peripheral arthritis [35]. In summary, the traditional therapies, including non-biological DMARDs, NSAIDs, and corticosteroids, do not adequately control disease activity in most patients who have severe disease [36]. In particular, there are no non-biological DMARDs that have proven to be efficacious for axial disease.

Clinical trials of etanercept

TNF-α is expressed in inflamed sacroiliac joints [37] synovium [38, 39] and serum [40, 41] of AS patients. Several RCTs have been performed and showed beneficial effects of etanercept in patients with AS [36, 42, 43]. The first pivotal (pilot) study in AS was a small RCT conducted in northern California [42]. Inclusion criteria required 1) definite AS by modified New York clinical criteria [44], 2) evidence of active spondylitis despite accepted treatments, 3) age at least 18 years old. Patients were excluded if they had a spondylitis other than AS, clinical or radiological evidence of complete spinal ankylosis, a history of recurrent infections or cancer, or a serious liver, renal, hematologic, or neurologic disorder. A total of 40 patients, predominantly Caucasian male, with long standing, persistently active disease, were randomized to etanercept (25 mg subcutaneously twice weekly) *versus* placebo injections for 4 months. In this study, a 20% or greater improvement in composite index (20% change in at least three of five measures which were: duration of morning stiffness, degree of nocturnal spinal pain, the Bath AS Functional Index, the patient's global assessment of disease activity, and the score for joint swelling) was the primary endpoint for the evaluation. A total of 80% of etanercept-treated patients achieved this treatment response *versus* 30% of placebo-treated patients ($p < 0.004$). Among the secondary outcome measures (physician's global assessment of disease activity, measure of spinal mobility measuring chest expansion, the scores for enthesitis, number of tender joints, ESR (erythrocyte sedimentation rate), and CRP (C-reactive protein), the observed changes favored the etanercept treatment group. Spinal mobility, as measured by the modified Schober's index and mean occiput-to-wall distance, was not significantly changed.

The second pivotal study was an international multi-center RCT which confirmed the efficacy of etanercept [36]. Inclusion criteria were generally similar to the pilot study. A total of 277 patients were randomized to etanercept (25 mg subcutaneously twice weekly) *versus* placebo. In this study, the Assessments in AS 20% response (ASAS20) [45] at 12 weeks was the primary endpoint for the evaluation. A total of 59% of etanercept-treated patients achieved an ASAS20 response *versus* 28% of placebo-treated patients ($p < 0.0001$) and by 57% and 22% of patients, respectively, at week 24 ($p < 0.0001$). All individual ASAS components, acute phase reactant levels, and spinal mobility measures were also significantly improved.

The third pivotal study was a multi-center RCT from Europe [43]. Of 84 patients (45 received etanercept and 39 received placebo), significant more etanercept patients than placebo patients (60% *versus* 23%, $p < 0.001$) were ASAS20 responders at week 12, the primary efficacy end point. Notably, significant improvements in the etanercept group were evident by week 2, the earliest assessment point, and were sustained thereafter.

These studies suggest that etanercept reduces the clinical signs and symptoms of AS and improve quality of life. Further research is needed to assess the longer-term effects of etanercept in patients with AS. Imaging study (e.g., magnetic resonance imaging –MRI) may also be helpful in determining the effect of etanercept on structural damage in these patients [46].

Conclusions

Robust efficacy results have been demonstrated for etanercept in patients with rheumatoid arthritis, psoriatic arthritis, juvenile rheumatoid arthritis and ankylosing spondylitis. The safety of etanercept is discussed elsewhere. Etanercept therapy represents a rational, mechanism-based targeted approach to the treatment of rheumatic diseases for which the cytokine TNF-α plays an important role.

References

1 Feldmann M, Maini RN (2001) Anti-TNF alpha therapy of rheumatoid arthritis: what have we learned? *Annu Rev Immunol* 19: 163–196

2 Gottlieb AB (2004) Etanercept for the treatment of psoriasis and psoriatic arthritis. *Dermatol Ther* 17(5): 401–408

3 Keller C, Webb A, Davis J (2003) Cytokines in the seronegative spondyloarthropathies and their modification by TNF blockade: a brief report and literature review. *Ann Rheum Dis* 62(12): 1128–1132

4 Grom AA, Murray KJ, Luyrink L, Emery H, Passo MH, Glass DN, Bowlin T, Edwards C 3rd (1996) Patterns of expression of tumor necrosis factor alpha, tumor necrosis factor beta, and their receptors in synovia of patients with juvenile rheumatoid arthritis and juvenile spondyloarthropathy. *Arthritis Rheum* 39(10): 1703–1710

5 Hochberg MC (1981) Adult and juvenile rheumatoid arthritis: current epidemiologic concepts. *Epidemiol Rev* 3: 27–44

6 Wolfe F, Mitchell DM, Sibley JT, Fries JF, Bloch DA, Williams CA, Spitz PW, Haga M, Kleinheksel SM, Cathey MA (1994) The mortality of rheumatoid arthritis. *Arthritis Rheum* 37(4): 481–494
7 Prior P, Symmons DP, Scott DL, Brown R, Hawkins CF (1984) Cause of death in rheumatoid arthritis. *Br J Rheumatol* 23(2): 92–99
8 Gridley G, McLaughlin JK, Ekbom A, Klareskog L, Adami HO, Hacker DG, Hoover R, Fraumeni JF (1993) Incidence of cancer among patients with rheumatoid arthritis. *J Natl Cancer Inst* 85(4): 307–311
9 Mellemkjaer L, Linet MS, Gridley G, Frisch M, Moller H, Olsen JH (1996) Rheumatoid arthritis and cancer risk. *Eur J Cancer* 32A(10): 1753–1757
10 Moreland LW, Baumgartner SW, Schiff MH, Schiff MH, Tindall EA, Fleischmann RM, Weaver AL, Ettlinger RE, Cohen S, Koopman WJ et al (1997) Treatment of rheumatoid arthritis with a recombinant human tumor necrosis factor receptor (p75)-Fc fusion protein. *N Engl J Med* 337(3): 141–147
11 Moreland LW, Schiff MH, Baumgartner SW, Tindall EA, Fleischmann RM, Bulpitt KJ, Weaver AL, Keystone EC, Furst DE, Mease PJ et al (1999) Etanercept therapy in rheumatoid arthritis. A randomized, controlled trial. *Ann Intern Med* 130(6): 478–486
12 Bathon JM, Martin RW, Fleischmann RM, Tesser JR, Schiff MH, Keystone EC, Genovese MC, Wasko MC, Moreland LW, Weaver AL et al (2000) A comparison of etanercept and methotrexate in patients with early rheumatoid arthritis. *N Engl J Med* 343(22): 1586–1593
13 Weinblatt ME, Kremer JM, Bankhurst AD, Bulpitt KJ, Fleischmann RM, Fox RI, Jackson CG, Lange M, Burge DJ et al (1999) A trial of etanercept, a recombinant tumor necrosis factor receptor:Fc fusion protein, in patients with rheumatoid arthritis receiving methotrexate. *N Engl J Med* 340(4): 253–259
14 Klareskog L, van der Heijde D, de Jager JP, Gough A, Kalden J, Malaise M, Martin, Mola E, Pavelka K, Sany J et al (2004) Therapeutic effect of the combination of etanercept and methotrexate compared with each treatment alone in patients with rheumatoid arthritis: double-blind randomised controlled trial. *Lancet* 363(9410): 675–681
15 Taylor WJ (2002) Epidemiology of psoriatic arthritis. *Curr Opin Rheumatol* 14(2): 98–103
16 Mease PJ, Goffe BS, Metz J, VanderStoep A, Finck B, Burge DJ (2000) Etanercept in the treatment of psoriatic arthritis and psoriasis: a randomised trial. *Lancet* 356(9227): 385–390
17 Mease PJ, Kivitz AJ, Burch FX, Siegel EL, Cohen SB, Ory P, Salonen D, Rubenstein J, Sharp JT, Tsuji W (2004) Etanercept treatment of psoriatic arthritis: safety, efficacy, and effect on disease progression. *Arthritis Rheum* 50(7): 2264–2272
18 Peterson LS, Mason T, Nelson AM, O'Fallon WM, Gabriel SE (1996) Juvenile rheumatoid arthritis in Rochester, Minnesota 1960–1993. Is the epidemiology changing? *Arthritis Rheum* 39(8): 1385–1390
19 Petty RE, Malleson P (1987) Epidemiology of juvenile rheumatoid arthritis. *World Pediatr Child Care* 3: 205–210
20 Ansell BM (1999) Prognosis in juvenile arthritis. *Adv Exp Med Biol* 455: 27–33
21 Andersson Gare B (1999) Juvenile arthritis—who gets it, where and when? A review of current data on incidence and prevalence. *Clin Exp Rheumatol* 17(3): 367–374
22 Prieur AM, Le Gall E, Karman F, Edan C, Lasserre O, Goujard J (1987) Epidemiologic survey of juvenile chronic arthritis in France. Comparison of data obtained from two different regions. *Clin Exp Rheumatol* 5(3): 217–223
23 Moe N, Rygg M (1998) Epidemiology of juvenile chronic arthritis in northern Norway: a ten-year retrospective study. *Clin Exp Rheumatol* 16(1): 99–101
24 Petty RE, Southwood TR, Baum J, Bhettay E, Glass DN, Manners P, Maldonado-Cocco J, Suarez-Almazor M, Orozco-Alcala J, Prieur AM (1998) Revision of the proposed classification criteria for juvenile idiopathic arthritis: Durban, 1997. *J Rheumatol* 25(10): 1991–1994
25 Lovell DJ, Giannini EH, Reiff A, Cawkwell GD, Silverman ED, Nocton JJ, Stein LD, Gedalia A, Ilowite NT, Wallace CA et al (2000) Etanercept in children with polyarticular juvenile rheumatoid arthritis. Pediatric Rheumatology Collaborative Study Group. *N Engl J Med* 342(11): 763–769
26 Lovell DJ, Giannini EH, Reiff A, Jones OY, Schneider R, Olson JC, Stein LD, Gedalia A, Ilowite NT, Wallace CA et al., Pediatric Rheumatology Collaborative Study Group (2003) Long-term efficacy and safety of etanercept in children with polyarticular-course juvenile rheumatoid arthritis: interim results from an ongoing multicenter, open-label, extended-treatment trial. *Arthritis Rheum* 48(1): 218–226

27 Quartier P, Taupin P, Bourdeaut F, Lemelle I, Pillet P, Bost M, Sibilia J, Kone-Paut I, Gandon-Laloum S, LeBideau M et al (2003) Efficacy of etanercept for the treatment of juvenile idiopathic arthritis according to the onset type. *Arthritis Rheum* 48(4): 1093–1101

28 Braun J, Bollow M, Remlinger G, Eggens U, Rudwaleit M, Distler A, Sieper J (1998) Prevalence of spondylarthropathies in HLA-B27 positive and negative blood donors. *Arthritis Rheum* 41(1): 58–67

29 Gran JT, Husby G, Hordvik M (1985) Prevalence of ankylosing spondylitis in males and females in a young middle-aged population of Tromso, northern Norway. *Ann Rheum Dis* 44(6): 359–367

30 Braun J, Sieper J (2002) Therapy of ankylosing spondylitis and other spondyloarthritides: established medical treatment, anti-TNF-alpha therapy and other novel approaches. *Arthritis Res* 4(5): 307–321

31 Lawrence RC, Helmick CG, Arnett FC, Deyo RA, Felson DT, Giannini EH, Heyse SP, Hirsch R, Hochberg MC, Hunder GG et al (1998) Estimates of the prevalence of arthritis and selected musculoskeletal disorders in the United States. *Arthritis Rheum* 41(5): 778–799

32 Baron M, Zendel I (1989) HLA-B27 testing in ankylosing spondylitis: an analysis of the pretesting assumptions. *J Rheumatol* 16(5): 631–634

33 Zink A, Braun J, Listing J, Wollenhaupt J (2000) Disability and handicap in rheumatoid arthritis and ankylosing spondylitis – results from the German rheumatological database. German Collaborative Arthritis Centers. *J Rheumatol* 27(3): 613–622

34 Leirisalo-Repo M (1998) Prognosis, course of disease, and treatment of the spondyloarthropathies. *Rheum Dis Clin North Am* 24(4): 737–751

35 Sampaio-Barros PD, Costallat LT, Bertolo MB, Neto JF, Samara AM (2000) Methotrexate in the treatment of ankylosing spondylitis. *Scand J Rheumatol* 29(3): 160–162

36 Davis JC Jr, Van Der Heijde D, Braun J, Dougados M, Cush J, Clegg DO, Kivitz A, Fleischmann R, Inman R, Tsuji W, Enbrel Ankylosing Spondylitis Study Group (2003) Recombinant human tumor necrosis factor receptor (etanercept) for treating ankylosing spondylitis: a randomized, controlled trial. *Arthritis Rheum* 48(11): 3230–3236

37 Braun J, Bollow M, Neure L, Seipelt E, Seyrekbasan F, Herbst H, Eggens U, Distler A, Sieper J (1995) Use of immunohistologic and *in situ* hybridization techniques in the examination of sacroiliac joint biopsy specimens from patients with ankylosing spondylitis. *Arthritis Rheum* 38(4): 499–505

38 Grom AA, Murray KJ, Luyrink L, Emery H, Passo MH, Glass DN, Bowlin T, Edwards C 3rd (1996) Patterns of expression of tumor necrosis factor alpha, tumor necrosis factor beta, and their receptors in synovia of patients with juvenile rheumatoid arthritis and juvenile spondyloarthropathy. *Arthritis Rheum* 39(10): 1703–1710

39 Canete JD, Llena J, Collado A, Sanmarti R, Gaya A, Gratacos J, Blay M, Munoz-Gomez J (1997) Comparative cytokine gene expression in synovial tissue of early rheumatoid arthritis and seronegative spondyloarthropathies. *Br J Rheumatol* 36(1): 38–42

40 Gratacos J, Collado A, Filella X, Sanmarti R, Canete J, Llena J, Molina R, Ballesta A, Munoz-Gomez J (1994) Serum cytokines (IL-6, TNF-alpha, IL-1 beta and IFN-gamma) in ankylosing spondylitis: a close correlation between serum IL-6 and disease activity and severity. *Br J Rheumatol* 33(10): 927–931

41 Toussirot E, Lafforgue P, Boucraut J, Despieds P, Schiano A, Bernard D, Acquaviva PC (1994) Serum levels of interleukin 1-beta, tumor necrosis factor-alpha, soluble interleukin 2 receptor and soluble CD8 in seronegative spondyloarthropathies. *Rheumatol Int* 13(5): 175–180

42 Gorman JD, Sack KE, Davis JC Jr, (2002) Treatment of ankylosing spondylitis by inhibition of tumor necrosis factor alpha. *N Engl J Med* 346(18): 1349–1356

43 Calin A, Dijkmans BA, Emery P, Hakala M, Kalden J, Leirisalo-Repo M, Mola EM, Salvarani C, Sanmarti R, Sany J et al (2004) Outcomes of a multicentre randomised clinical trial of etanercept to treat ankylosing spondylitis. *Ann Rheum Dis* 63(12): 1594–1600

44 van der Linden S, Valkenburg HA, Cats A (1984) Evaluation of diagnostic criteria for ankylosing spondylitis. A proposal for modification of the New York criteria. *Arthritis Rheum* 27(4): 361–368

45 Anderson JJ, Baron G, van der Heijde D, Felson DT, Dougados M (2001) Ankylosing spondylitis assessment group preliminary definition of short-term improvement in ankylosing spondylitis. *Arthritis Rheum* 44(8): 1876–1886

46 Baraliakos X, Davis J, Tsuji W, Braun J (2005) Magnetic resonance imaging examinations of the spine in patients with ankylosing spondylitis before and after therapy with the tumor necrosis factor alpha receptor fusion protein etanercept. *Arthritis Rheum* 52(4): 1216–1223

TNF-alpha Inhibitors
Edited by Jeffrey M. Weinberg and Robin Buchholz

Etanercept in dermatology and off-label use

Noah Gratch[1] and Andrew F. Alexis[2]

[1] *Joan and Sanford Weill Medical College of Cornell University, New York, NY 10021, USA*
[2] *St. Luke's-Roosevelt Hospital, 1090 Amsterdam Avenue Suite 11B, New York, NY 10025, USA*

Introduction

The first biologic tumor necrosis factor (TNF-α) inhibitor to be approved for dermatologic use is etanercept. Etanercept is a fusion protein that consists of the extracellular portion of the TNF-α receptor linked to the Fc portion of human IgG. By binding to soluble and cell membrane bound TNF-α, it is effective in the treatment of TNF-mediated inflammatory diseases of the skin and other organ systems. In the USA etanercept has been approved by the Food and Drug Administration (FDA) for use in rheumatoid arthritis (since 1998), psoriatic arthritis (since 2002), ankylosing spondylitis (since 2003), psoriasis (since 2004), and in juvenile rheumatoid arthritis (since 2000). The use of etanercept as an approved and off-label therapeutic in dermatology is evaluated in this chapter.

Etanercept in psoriasis and psoriatic arthritis

Psoriasis is an idiopathic chronic inflammatory disease that is characterized by scaly, erythematous plaques on the skin. Involvement of the joints, psoriatic arthritis (PsA), occurs in an estimated 7–42% of psoriasis patients and can contribute significantly to the morbidity of the disease [1]. TNF-α has been implicated in the pathogenesis of psoriasis and psoriatic arthritis. In psoriasis, TNF-α induces keratinocyte hyperproliferation and production of proinflammatory cytokines [2, 3]. TNF-α expression is increased in the stratum corneum of psoriatic lesions compared to uninvolved skin [4]. In addition, increased serum levels of TNF-α have been demonstrated in psoriatic patients [5]. There is elevated TNF-α production in psoriatic lesional skin as compared to uninvolved skin from healthy volunteers [4]. Furthermore, serum and lesional levels of TNF-α correlate with improvement in psoriasis while a decrease in TNF-α levels paralleled a clinical improvement in treated patients [5, 6].

Psoriatic arthritis (PsA) is a destructive seronegative arthropathy characterized by asymmetric inflammation and joint destruction. Variable involvement of axial and interphalangeal joints, tenosynovitis, dactylitis, and enthesopathy are characteristic features. Psoriasis (of the skin) typically precedes the onset of psoriatic arthritis and it is therefore often first diagnosed by dermatologists [1]. TNF-α appears to be an important mediator of psoriatic arthritis; high levels of TNF-α have been demonstrated in PsA joint fluid and synovium compared to osteoarthritis controls [7].

Etanercept has been approved for reducing signs and symptoms and inhibiting the progression of structural damage of active arthritis in PsA. The safety and efficacy of etanercept in the treatment of psoriatic arthritis was investigated in a number of randomized clinical trials [8, 9] and is discussed in detail in Chapter 4.

Inhibition of TNF-α has also been shown to be a safe and effective strategy in the treatment of psoriasis [8–11]. In a Phase II randomized, placebo-controlled study, Gottlieb et al. [12] demonstrated the efficacy and safety of etanercept 25 mg BIW in the treatment of moderate to severe plaque psoriasis. Selected patients were 18 years of age or older, and had prior systemic therapy or phototherapy for psoriasis (including psoralen plus UV-A, UV-B, oral retinoids, cyclosporine, or methotrexate). Patients with guttate, erythrodermic, or pustular psoriasis were excluded. All systemic therapies including psoralen and UV-A were stopped a month prior to treatment, and UV-B and topical therapies, excluding mild topical steroids and shampoos to the scalp, axilla, and groin, were not allowed 2 weeks prior to baseline measurements. The primary endpoint for efficacy in psoriasis was measured using the Psoriasis Area and Severity Index (PASI). This is a 72-point scale that evaluates area of involvement and the erythema, induration, and desquamation of these areas. PASI 75 was the primary endpoint for measuring psoriasis at 12 weeks. In this 24 week study of 112 patients, PASI 75 was achieved in 30% and 56% of patients at weeks 12 and 24, compared to 2% and 5% in the placebo group, respectively (Fig. 1). No opportunistic infections were seen and no serious adverse events

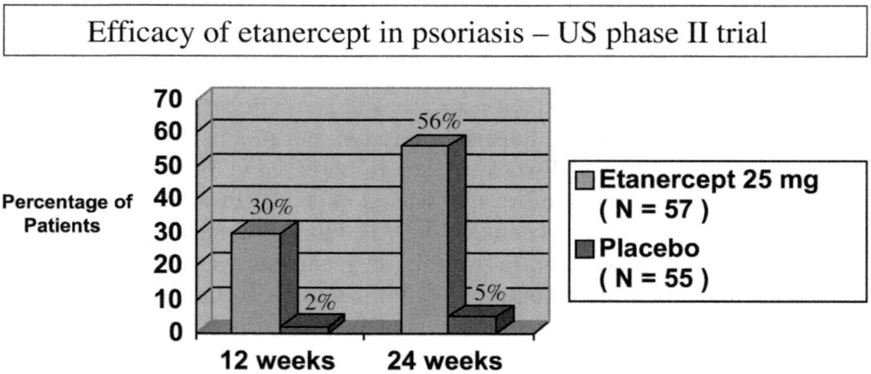

Figure 1. Percentage of psoriatic patients achieving PASI 75 with etanercept 25 mg BIW or placebo [12].

were considered to be directly related to etanercept; only injection site reactions were more common in the etanercept group as compared to the placebo group.

Two large Phase III trials have evaluated etanercept in the treatment of moderate to severe psoriasis, one in the US [13] and one international study involving sites in the US, Canada, and Western Europe [14]. Both trials were double-blinded, randomized, placebo-controlled studies. As seen in the Phase II study, clinical improvement continued to improve with longer treatment and, in these studies, an accelerated rate of improvement was seen in higher dose treatment groups. In the US study, eligibility criteria were similar to those in the Phase II study; however, patients who had prior biological therapy were excluded. Of 672 patients, 652 patients were randomized to receive placebo, etanercept 25 mg once a week (low-dose, N = 160) or twice a week (medium-dose, N = 162), or etanercept 50 mg twice a week (high-dose, N = 164). Placebo patients were crossed over at Week 12 to receive etanercept 25 mg BIW. The proportion of patients who achieved PASI 75 correlated with increasing dose and duration of treatment, 14%, 34%, and 49% in the low-dose, medium-dose, and high dose groups, respectively, compared to 4% in the placebo group at Week 12 ($P < 0.001$). At 24 weeks, PASI 75 was 25% in the low-dose, 44% in the medium dose, and 59% in the high dose groups (Tab. 1). A statistically significant difference in the mean percentage of improvement, as measured by PASI, was seen in all three etanercept groups as early as 2 weeks. Likewise, improvement in patients' global assessment and quality of life as measured by Dermatology Life Quality Index (DLQI) became statistically significant at 2 weeks and continued for the duration of the study. There was a favorable safety profile and the number of patients reporting adverse events and infection were similar in etanercept and placebo groups. No tuberculosis or opportunistic infections were recorded during the studies. No severe laboratory abnormalities in hematologic analysis, serum chemistry and urinalysis were noted and no patients withdrew because of an

Table 1. Clinical response of etanercept on psoriasis improvement as measured by percentage improvement of PASI

	Clinical response of etanercept treatment on psoriasis: US phase III trial					
	12 Weeks			24 Weeks		
	PASI 50	PASI 75	PASI 90	PASI 50	PASI 75	PASI 90
Placebo N = 166	14	4	1	NP	33	NP
Low dose N = 160	41	14	3	58	25	6
Medium dose N = 162	58	34	12	70	44	20
High dose N = 164	74	49	22	77	59	30

Treatment groups: placebo, low dose treatment group (25 mg once a week) medium dose (25 mg BIW), and high dose group (50 mg BIW). NP = not provided [13].

abnormal laboratory value. Screening for anti-etanercept antibodies in all etanercept treated patients, performed at 24 weeks, detected 8 patients who had developed non-neutralizing antibodies. The authors did not observe a difference in the adverse-events profiles and efficacy outcomes between the eight patients who had developed antibodies and the patients without anti-etanercept antibodies. At 6 months, patients who achieved PASI 75 discontinued treatment with etanercept. Upon withdrawal there were no flares or rebounds of psoriasis reported. The mean duration of PASI 75, following withdrawal, was 1–2 months [15].

In the international study evaluating etanercept at medium-dose (25 mg BIW) and high-dose (50 mg BIW), faster improvement was seen in patients who received higher dose etanercept. All patients including the placebo, medium dose, and high dose groups were treated with etanercept 25 mg BIW after 12 weeks, in order to evaluate if the benefit gained by the higher dose etanercept, as shown by Leonardi et al. [13], was maintained when the dose was reduced to 25 mg twice a week. Of the 91 patients in the high-dose group who had achieved PASI 75 at 12 weeks, 77% (70/91) maintained PASI 75 at 24 weeks. All treatment groups showed improved PASI scores over the second half of the study (Fig. 2). Similar to previous trials, etanercept was well tolerated, and, outside of an increase in injection site reactions in the etanercept group during the first 12 weeks, the frequency of adverse events and infections was similar in all groups over the course of the study [14]. Based on this study the FDA has approved the dosing of etanercept for psoriasis treatment at 50 mg BIW for the first 12 weeks followed thereafter by 25 mg BIW.

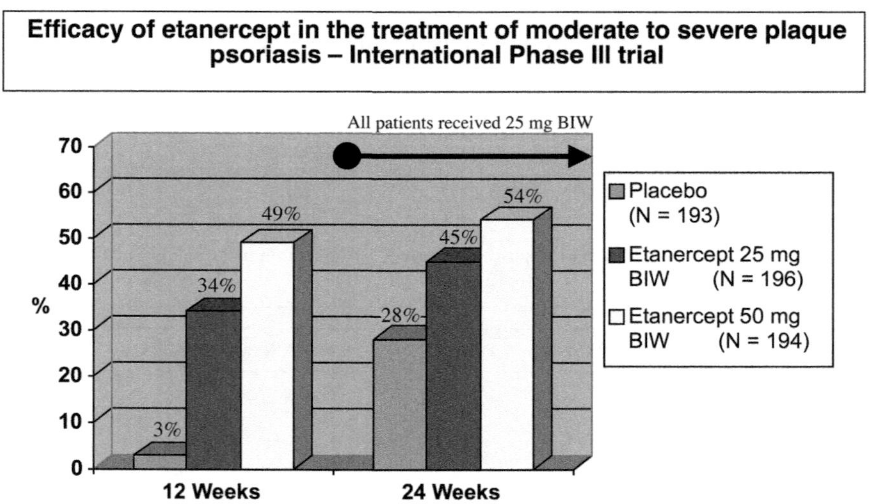

Figure 2. Percentage of psoriasis patients achieving PASI 75 at 12 weeks in placebo, low dose and high dose groups; and at 24 weeks after all groups were treated with etanercept 25 mg BIW [14].

Off-label use of etanercept in dermatology

Given the important role of TNF-α in the pathophysiology of inflammatory skin diseases other than psoriasis, a growing number of off-label uses of etanercept have been reported. Investigation into potential off-label dermatologic uses is largely limited to case reports and small case series; however, a small number of clinical trials have been conducted. The majority of these reports involve patients with severe, recalcitrant disease which did not respond to standard therapy. Reported investigations include cicatricial pemphigoid [16], pemphigus vulgaris [17], pemphigus vulgaris and pemphigus vegetans [18], Langerhan's cell histiocytosis [19], SAPHO syndrome [20], Hyperimmunoglobulinemia D and Periodic Fever Syndrome [21], Churg-Straus-Syndrome [22], PAPA syndrome [23], multicentric reticulohistiocytosis [24], silicone granulomas [25], common variable immunodeficiency [26], apthous stomatitis [27], pyoderma gangrenosum [28], and subacute cutaneous lupus erythematosus [29].

Randomized and open clinical trials of etanercept in the treatment of Behçet's, Still's disease, cutaneous T-cell lymphoma (CTCL), sarcoid, systemic sclerosis, and graft-*versus*-host-disease (GVHD) have been reported. These will be reviewed below.

Behçet's is an idiopathic inflammatory disease characterized by painful oral and genital ulcerations, arthritis, uveititis, cerebritits, erythema nodosum, and pustular skin eruptions. Increased TNF-α levels in the serum and in the aqueous humor of Behçet's patients with active disease have been reported, implicating TNF-α a central role in its pathogenesis [30]. In a double-blind, placebo controlled trial with etanercept 25 mg or placebo, twice a week, was administered to 40 male patients with Behçet's disease over a 4 week period [31]. All patients, except two in the etanercept group and one in the control (azathioprine or corticosteroids), underwent a 4 week washout period with prior treatments. In this short, small trial etanercept did not suppress pathergy or skin hyperactivity, but it allowed a significant reduction in oral ulcers, papulopustular lesions, and nodular lesions. This benefit from etanercept was not maintained after etanercept was withdrawn, and there was a significant worsening of arthritis in the etanercept group at 3 months post treatment.

A role for TNF-α inhibition in the treatment of Still's disease, an inflammatory disorder associated with fever, transient rash and joint pain or arthritis, has been inferred from previous successful use of thalidomide, which is known to reduce levels of TNF-α mRNA [32]. In a 6-month open trial of etanercept (25 mg, twice a week) and concomitant therapies (prednisone, methotrexate [MTX], and non-steroidal anti-inflammatory drugs [NSAIDS]), some efficacy was seen [33]. 12 patients, all with active arthritis, were enrolled and 10 completed the study. Two patients withdrew secondary to flare of fever, rash and arthritis. Of the 10 patients who completed the trial, seven showed improvement of arthritis. In an observational study of TNF-α agents in patients with refractory adult Still's disease, 10 of 20 patients who had received etanercept in combination with disease-modifying antirheumatic drugs and prednisone showed only partial remission of either arthritis, rash, myalgia and fever [34].

A pilot study in cutaneous T-cell lymphoma (CTCL) suggests there may be a role for etanercept in early disease management [35]. Etanercept 25 mg BIW was used in 12 patients (Stage I–IIA, 3 patients; Stage IIB–IV, 9 patients) who had failed prior treatments (α-interferon, total body electron beam, multiagent chemotherapy, retinoids, and topical nitrogen mustard therapy). Only two patients with early disease (Stage IB) showed improvement; one patient had a partial response and the other had a minor response. There was no response seen in patients with advanced, refractory disease.

Sarcoidosis is an idiopathic multisystem granulomatous disease affecting the skin, lungs, and many internal organs. Implication of increased TNF-α production by alveolar macrophages in pulmonary sarcoid prompted a Phase II trial of etanercept [36]. This Phase II trial of etanercept in progressive pulmonary sarcoidosis was terminated early due to treatment failure. Despite the lack of efficacy in progressive pulmonary sarcoidosis, there is a reported case relating cutaneous improvement with etanercept [37]. The patient had chronic sarcoidosis affecting the lungs, joints and skin and was poorly responsive to prednisone, methotrexate, and hydroxychloroquine. Addition of etanercept 25 mg twice weekly allowed discontinuation of prednisone and hydroxychloroquine, reduction of methotrexate, and clinical quiescence of her disease, including noted improved skin findings.

Systemic sclerosis is a progressive connective tissue disorder characterized by fibrosis of the skin and other internal organs. The potential use of TNF-α blockade in treating diffuse systemic sclerosis was evaluated in a pilot study [38]. 10 patients were treated with 25 mg, twice a week for 6 months. The results were encouraging in that four patients had improved skin scores; three of four patients with digital ulcerations had improvement, while pulmonary function remained stable.

Graft-*versus*-host-disease (GVHD) is an immunologic reaction in which donor immunocompetent T cells cause end organ damage in an allogenic host incapable of rejecting them [39]. Similar to systemic sclerosis, GVHD in its chronic form can lead to a fibrosis of the skin and involve other organs systems as well [39]. Studies in lethal GVHD mice models have shown a protective effect given by anti-TNF-α antibodies [40]. The use of etanercept in 10 chronic GVHD patients in combination with prednisone showed a favorable improvement in seven patients and allowed steroid tapering in half of the patients [41].

Although there is substantial evidence to support etanercept in treating moderate to severe plaque psoriasis, clinical trials have excluded patients with guttate, pustular and erythrodermic forms. A pustular flare, triggered by cyclosporine withdrawal, improved after brief treatment with etanercept, although residual erythema remained [42]. Palmoplantar psoriasis, a protean form of psoriasis, is not addressed in the previous studies. Weinberg reported a case of recalcitrant palmoplantar psoriasis, which responded with near total clearance after 5 months of etanercept [43].

Conclusion

In the 7 years of clinical follow-up and post marketing experience, over 280,000 patients worldwide have been treated with etanercept [44]. Overall, there has been a sustained efficacy and safety, and a favorable risk–benefit profile. In blinded, controlled trials in psoriasis and psoriatic arthritis adverse events between etanercept and placebo were comparable and there were no serious adverse events. The most common adverse effect was injection site reactions that were seen in 17% of patients. The reactions were described as mild to moderate, and tended to decrease in frequency after the first month of therapy [15]. Considerable safety and efficacy were seen in these controlled studies of 6 months duration, though further long-term evaluation in psoriasis and psoriatic arthritis is warranted.

Preliminary investigations have shown potential for etanercept as treatment in other dermatologic conditions. Further controlled studies and research will help establish the potential role and the limitations of etanercept in dermatology. The chronic nature of most dermatologic disease poses a considerable clinical challenge when considering the long-term safety of biologic agents, including etanercept. A detailed discussion on the safety of etanercept and other TNF-α inhibitors is included in Chapter 10.

References

1 Gladman DD (1998) Psoriatic arthritis. In: PJ Maddison, DA Isenberg, P Woo, DN Glass (eds): *Oxford Textbook of Rheumatology*. Oxford University Press, 1071
2 Bonifati C, Ameglio F (1999) Cytokines in Psoriasis. *Int J Dermatol* 38: 241–251
3 Yamauchi PS, Gindi V, Lowe NJ (2004) The treatment of psoriasis and psoriatic arthritis with etanercept: practical considerations on monotherapy, combination therapy, and safety. *Dermatol Clin* 22: 449–459
4 Ettehadi P, Greaves WM, Wallach D, Aderka D, Camp RDR (1994) Elevated tumor necrosis factor-α (TNF-α) biological activity in psoriatic skin lesions. *Clin Exp Immunol* 96: 146–151
5 Bonifati C, Carducci M, Cordial Fei P, Trento E, Sacerdoti G, Fazio M, Ameglio F (1994) Correlated increases of tumor necrosis factor-α, interleukin-6 and granulocyte monocyte-colony stimulating factor levels in suction blister fluids and sera of psoriatic patients – relationships with disease activity. *Clin Exp Derm atoll* 19: 383–387
6 Mussi A, Bonifati C, Carducci M, D'Agosto G, Pimpinelli F, D'Urso D, D'Auria L, Fazio M, Ameglio F (1997) Serum TNF-α levels correlate with disease severity and are reduced by effective therapy in plaque-type psoriasis. *J Biol Regul Homeost Agents* 11: 115–118
7 Partsch G, Steiner G, Leeb BF, Dunky F, Broll H, Smolen JS (1997) Highly increased levels of tumor necrosis factor-alpha and other proinflammatory cytokines in psoriatic arthritis synovial fluid. *J Rheumatol* 24(3): 518–523
8 Mease PJ, Goffe BS, Metz J, Vanderstoep A, Finck B, Burge DJ (2000) Etanercept in the treatment of psoriatic arthritis and psoriasis: a randomized trial. *Lancet* 356: 385–390
9 Mease PJ, Kivitz AJ, Burch FX, Siegel EL, Cohen SB, Ory B, Salonen D, Rubenstein J, Sharp JT,

Tsuji W (2004) Etanercept Treatment of Psoriatic Arthritis. *Arthritis Rheum* 50 (7): 2264–2272
10 Oh CJ, Das KM, Gottlieb AB (2000) Treatment with anti-tumor necrosis factor a (TNF-α) monoclonal antibody dramatically decreases the clinical activity of psoriasis lesions. *J Am Acad Dermatol* 42: 829–830
11 Chaudhari U, Romano P, Mulcahy LD, Dooley LT, Baker DG, Gottlieb AB (2001) Efficacy and safety of infliximab monotherapy for plaque-type psoriasis: a randomized trial. *Lancet* 357: 1842–1847
12 Gottleib AB, Matheson RT, Lowe N, Krueger GG, Kang S, Goffe BS, Gaspari A, Ling M, Weinstein GD, Nayak A et al (2003) A randomized trial of etanercept as monotherapy for psoriasis. *Arch Dermatol* 139: 1627–1632
13 Leonardi CL, Powers JL, Matheson RT, Goffe BS, Zitnik R, Wang A, Gottlieb AB (2003) Etanercept as monotherapy in patients with psoriasis. *N Engl J Med* 349: 2014–2022
14 Papp KA, Tyring S, Lahfa M, Prinz J, Griffiths CEM, Nakanishi AM, Zitnick R, van de Kerkhof PCM (2005) A global phase III randomized controlled trial of etanercept in psoriasis: safety, efficacy, and effect of dose reduction. *Br J Dermatol* 152: 1304–1312
15 Enbrel [package insert]. Thousand Oaks (CA). Amgen 2004
16 Sacher C, Rubbert A, König C, Scharffetter-Kochanek K, Kreig T, Hunzelmann N (2002) Treatment of recalcitrant cicatricial pemphigoid with the tumor necrosis factor α antagonist etanercept. *J Am Acad Dermatol* 46: 113–115
17 Berookhim B, Fischer HD, Weinberg JM (2004) Treatment of recalcitrant Pemphigus vulgaris with the Tumor Necrosis Factor α Antagonist Etanercept. *Cutis* 74: 245–247
18 Lin M, Hsu C, Lee JY (2005) Successful treatment of recalcitrant pemphigus vulgaris and pemphigus vegetans with etanercept and carbon dioxide laser. *Arch Dermatol* 141: 680–682
19 Henter JI, Karlen J, Calming U, Bernstrand C, Andersson U, Fadeel B (2001) Successful treatment of Langerhans'-cell histiocytosis with etanercept. *N Engl J Med* 345: 1577–1578
20 Wagner AD, Andresen J, Jendro MC, Hulsemann JL, Zeidler H (2002) Sustained response to tumor necrosis factor α-blocking agents in two patients with SAPHO syndrome. *Arthritis Rheum* 46 (7): 1965–1968
21 Takada K, Aksentijevich I, Mahadevan V, Dean JA, Kelley RI, Kastner DL (2003) Favorable preliminary experience with etanercept in two patients with the hyperimmunoglobulinemia d and periodic fever syndrome. *Arthritis Rheum* 48 (9): 2645–2651
22 Arbach O, Gross WL, Gause A (2002) Treatment of refractory churg-strauss-syndrome by TNF-α blockade. *Immunobiol* 206: 496–501
23 Cortis E, De Benedetti F, Insalaco A, Cioschi S, Muratori F, D'Urbano LE, Ugazio AG (2004) abnormal production of the tumor necrosis factor inhibitor etanercept and clinical efficacy of tumor in a patient with PAPA syndrome. *J Pediatr* 145: 851–855
24 Kovach BT, Calamia KT, Walsh JS, Ginsburg WW (2004) Treatment of multicentric reticulohistiocytosis With etanercept. *Arch Dermatol* 140: 919–921
25 Pasternack FR, Fox LP, Engler DE (2005) silicone granulomas treated with etanercept. *Arch Dermatol* 141: 13–15
26 Smith KJ, Skelton H (2001) Common variable immunodeficiency treated with a recombinant human IgG, tumour necrosis factor-α receptor fusion protein. *Br J Dermatol* 144: 597–600
27 Robinson ND, Guitart J (2003) Recalcitrant, recurrent apthous stomatitis treated with etanercept. *Arch Dermatol* 139: 1259–1262
28 McGowan JW, Johnson CA, Lynn A (2004) Treatment of pyoderma gangrenosum with etanercept. *J Drugs Dermatol* 3(4): 441–444
29 Fautrel B, Foltz V, Frances C, Bourgeois P, Rozenberg S (2002) Regression of subacute lupus erythematosus in a patient with rheumatoid arthritis treated with a biologic tumor necrosis factor alpha-blocking agent: comment on the article by Pisetsky and the letter from Aringer et al *Arthritis Rheum* 46 (5): 1408–1409
30 Sfikakis PP (2002) Behçet's disease: a new target for anti-tumor necrosis factor treatment. *Ann Rheum Dis* 61(Supl II): ii51–ii53
31 Melikoglu M, Fresko I, Mat C, Ozyazgan Y, Gogus F, Yurdakul S, Hamuryudan V, Yazici H (2005) Short-term trial of etanercept in Behçet's disease: a double blind, placebo controlled study. *J Rheumatol* 32: 98–105
32 Stambe C, Wicks IP (1998) TNF-α and response of treatment-resistant adult-onset Still's disease to thalidomide. *Lancet* 352 (9127): 544–545
33 Husni ME, Maier AL, Mease PJ, Overman SS, Fraser P, Gravallese EM, Weinblatt ME (2002)

Etanercept in the Treatment of Adult Patients With Still's Disease. *Arthritis Rheum* 46 (5): 1171–1176
34 Fautrel B, Sibilia J, Mariette X, Combe B (2005) Tumor necrosis factor α blocking agents in refractory adult Still's disease: an observational study of 20 cases. *Ann Rheum Dis* 64: 262–266
35 Tsimberidou AM, Giles FJ, Duvic M, Kurzrock R (2004) Pilot study of etanercept in patients with relapsed cutaneous T-cell lymphomas. *J Am Acad Dermatol* 51: 200–204
36 Utz JP, Limper AH, Kalra S, Specks U, Scott JP, Vuk-Pavlovic Z, Schroeder DR (2003) Etanercept for the treatment of stage II and stage III progressive pulmonary sarcoidosis. *Chest* 124 (1): 177–185
37 Khanna D, Liebling MR, Louie JS (2003) Etanercept ameliorates sarcoidosis arthritis and skin disease. *J Rheumatol* 30: 1864–1847
38 Ellman MH, MacDonald PA, Hayes FA (2000) Etanercept as treatment for diffuse scleroderma: a pilot study. Abstract. *Arthritis Rheum* 43: S392
39 Penas PF, Fernandez-Herrera J, Garcia-Diez A (2004) Dermatologic treatment of cutaneous graft *versus* host disease. *Am J Clin Dermatol* 5(6): 403–416
40 Hattori K, Hirano T, Miyajima H, Yamakawa N, Tateno M, Oshimi K, Kayagaki N, Yagita H, Okumura K (1998) Differential effects of anti-fas ligand and anti-tumor necrosis factor α antibodies on acute graft-*versus*-host-disease pathologies. *Blood* 91 (11): 4051–4055
41 Chiang KY, Abhyankar S, Bridges K, Godder K, Henslee-Downey JP (2002) Recombinant human tumor necrosis factor receptor fusion protein as complimentary treatment for chronic graft-*versus*-host disease. *Transplantation* 73 (4): 665–667
42 Kamarashev J, Lor P, Forster A, Heinzerling L, Burg G, Nestle FO (2002) Generalized pustular psoriasis induced by cyclosporine a withdrawal responding to the tumor necrosis factor alpha inhibitor etanercept. *Dermatol* 205 (2): 213–216
43 Weinberg JM (2003) Successful treatment of recalcitrant palmoplantar psoriasis with etanercept. *Cutis* 72: 396–398
44 www.enbrel.com

TNF-alpha Inhibitors
Edited by Jeffrey M. Weinberg and Robin Buchholz

Infliximab in rheumatology

Mihaela B. Taylor and Dahlia T. Lainer

David Geffen School of Medicine, UCLA Medical Center, Los Angeles, CA 90095, USA

In recent years, the addition of therapeutic agents generated by recombinant or monoclonal antibody biotechnology has enhanced our armamentarium in treating autoimmune disorders. Targeting tumor necrosis factor-α (TNF-α) in disorders such as Crohn's disease, rheumatoid arthritis (RA), ankylosing spondylitis (AS), psoriatic arthritis (PsA) and psoriasis has had a major impact on symptom control and disease progression. This chapter attempts to provide a summary of infliximab uses in rheumatology. Infliximab has been approved by the US Food and Drug Administration (FDA) for treatment of RA, AS and PsA. However, the drug has also demonstrated promising benefits in a variety of other rheumatologic conditions, such as inflammatory myositis, giant cell arteritis, sarcoidosis and Behçet's disease.

Rheumatoid arthritis

Current understanding of RA pathogenesis attributes a pivotal role to TNF-α. Several findings strongly support this hypothesis. TNF-α was found to degrade cartilage and bone *in vitro*; additionally, it co-localizes with TNF receptors in RA synovium and the pannus-cartilage junction [1]. The molecule was shown to be vital in regulating the production of interleukin (IL)-1 in cultured RA-derived synovial cells (a mixture of lymphoid cells, macrophages, dendritic cells, B cells, endothelial cells, and fibroblasts) [2]. Finally, TNF-α was noted to have arthritogenic properties in animal models. Blocking TNF-α with monoclonal antibodies ameliorated disease in murine collagen induced arthritis (CIA), even when given after the onset of arthritis [3, 4]. The strongest evidence that TNF-α is indeed crucial to the pathogenesis of RA came with the first human application of cA2 in RA. cA2 is a chimeric human/mouse monoclonal anti-TNF-α antibody, consisting of the constant regions of human (Hu)IgG1κ, coupled to the Fv regions of a high affinity neutralizing murine anti-Hu TNF-α antibody (A2) [5, 6]. The antibody was produced by Centocor, Inc. and later named infliximab. Infliximab binds to soluble TNF-α as well as membrane bound TNF-α. It does not bind to TNF-β (lymphotoxin α). Because infliximab is a protein, it is not metabolized by cytochrome P-450 enzymes. This reduces the degree of individual patient variability with regard to toxic or inactive metabolites and diminishes the risk of complex drug interactions [7]. Infliximab has a primarily intravascular distribution. The terminal half life is 8–12 days with no accumulation of the drug by repeated dosing.

In 1993, Elliott et al. [5] used cA2 in an open label Phase I/II trial in 20 patients with active erosive RA that fulfilled ACR criteria for diagnosis and who had not adequately responded to disease modifying anti-rheumatic drugs (DMARDs). Patients received a total of 20 mg/kg of cA2 over 2 weeks. The study concluded that the molecule was safe and well-tolerated. Additionally, patients demonstrated significant clinical and laboratory improvement after 8 weeks. Prior to the publication of this study, therapeutic options for rheumatoid arthritis were toxic, non-specific and minimally effective. The important scientific breakthrough of this study was the realization that targeting a single cytokine *in vivo* could be safe, precise and successful.

The positive results of this study led to a dose-finding double-blind placebo-controlled trial that randomized 73 patients with active RA who had failed at least one DMARD to receive a single infusion of 1 mg/kg or 10 mg/kg of cA2 [8]. The primary endpoint was achievement of a Paulus 20 at week 4 [9]. The study found impressive immediate short-term results, with 79% of patients in the 10 mg/kg group achieving Paulus 20 and 58% of patients achieving Paulus 50, significantly better than placebo. The 1 mg/kg infusion was effective compared to placebo but provided less response than the higher dose group. Notably, C-reactive protein (CRP) rapidly decreased within 3 days of treatment.

Kavanaugh et al. conducted a dose-ranging study of infliximab in patients who were on stable doses of methotrexate (MTX) [10]. 28 patients were randomized to receive a single infusion of placebo or 5, 10, or 20 mg/kg of infliximab. Then, after completing the blinded portion of the study, 23 patients entered an open-label, repeated treatment extension phase in which they received up to three additional 10 mg/kg infusions at 8 week intervals. Primary endpoint was achievement of an ACR20 response [11]. In the blinded portion of the study, 81% (17/21) of patients who received infliximab achieved an ACR20 response, compared to 14.3% (1/7) of patients who received placebo. Responses were similar among the different infliximab dose groups. Interestingly, among patients who received infliximab during the blinded and open-label portions of the study, 53% maintained an ACR20 response through week 40.

A follow-up randomized double-blind placebo-controlled multicenter trial was conducted to determine the efficacy and optimal dose of infliximab. Additionally, it attempted to establish any enhanced therapeutic efficacy when co-administered with MTX [12]. The study enrolled 101 patients with active RA despite at least 6 months of MTX treatment to receive either MTX with placebo or MTX with infliximab 1 mg/kg, 3 mg/kg or 10 mg/kg given at weeks 0, 2, 6, 10 and 14. Patients were followed for 26 weeks and response was assessed by the Paulus criteria. Approximately 60% of patients receiving either 3 mg/kg or 10 mg/kg of infliximab with or without MTX achieved a Paulus 20 response. The duration of response in the 3 mg/kg and 10 mg/kg infliximab groups was significantly longer than that of the placebo group. Importantly, in the infliximab groups, duration of response was better sustained with concomitant MTX administration.

Long-term efficacy was demonstrated in a 2 year, double-blind, placebo-controlled international multicenter Anti-Tumor necrosis factor Trial in Rheumatoid Arthritis with Concomitant Therapy (ATTRACT) [13–16]. The study enrolled 428 patients with active RA despite MTX therapy. Patients' median age was 54 years, median disease duration was 8.4 years and median swollen and tender joint counts were 20 and 31, respectively. Patients had failed a median of 3 DMARDs and about 50% were in functional Class III. All patients received treatment with MTX and were randomized to one of five treatment groups: infliximab 3 mg/kg every 4 or 8 weeks, infliximab 10 mg/kg every 4 or 8 weeks, or placebo every 4 weeks. Infusions were administered at weeks 0, 2, and 6 with subsequent treatment based on their randomization schedule. Patients were treated for at least 2 years. The primary endpoint of ATTRACT was the achievement of ACR20 response by week 30; at 54 weeks, the prevention of progression of joint damage was assessed by the change from baseline in the modified Sharp/van der Heijde score (vdH-S) [17, 18]; at 102 weeks, the improvement in physical function was assessed by the health assessment questionnaire (HAQ) [19] and short form 36 health survey (SF-36) [20].

All doses of infliximab resulted in significant improvement as measured by the ACR20 through week 102 when compared to MTX alone – 43–52% of patients achieved a clinical response at 30 weeks compared with only 20% of MTX control patients (Tab. 1). This response rate was statistically significant for each infliximab dose group when compared to MTX alone and remained significant at weeks 54 and 102. Further, the 3 mg/kg every 8 weeks dosing schedule was as effective as the higher 10 mg/kg dose or the more frequent 4 week interval. Compared to patients treated with MTX alone, a significantly

Table 1. ATTRACT: Clinical response

	30 week analysis		54 week analysis		102 week analysis	
Parameter	All infliximab (n = 340)	Placebo (n = 88)	All infliximab (n = 340)	Placebo (n = 88)	All infliximab (n = 340)	Placebo (n = 88)
ACR20 Response	52%*	20%	52%*	17%	43%*	16%
ACR50 Response	28%*	5%	33%*	9%	27%*	6%
ACR70 Response	12%**	0	18%*	3%	15%*	1%

*$p < 0.001$ **$p = 0.003$

higher number of infliximab-treated patients achieved ACR50 (5% *versus* 28%) and ACR70 (0% *versus* 12%) responses. Treatment with infliximab was also associated with statistically significant improvement in tender joint pain, swollen joint count, and levels of inflammatory markers in the blood.

With regard to radiographic changes, among the 340 patients treated with infliximab, 259 had complete radiographs available for analysis. There was significant inhibition of structural damage progression (as measured by vdH-S) at weeks 54 and 102 compared to baseline in patients treated with infliximab (all doses) *versus* placebo (Tab. 2). There were no differences among the various infliximab groups. At week 102, additional endpoints were evaluated, including prevention of new erosions, as well as individual results of the two components of the vdH-S score, bone erosions and joint space narrowing. Patients treated with infliximab were found to have significantly fewer new erosions and less erosive damage than those treated with MTX alone.

Table 2. ATTRACT: Radiographic response

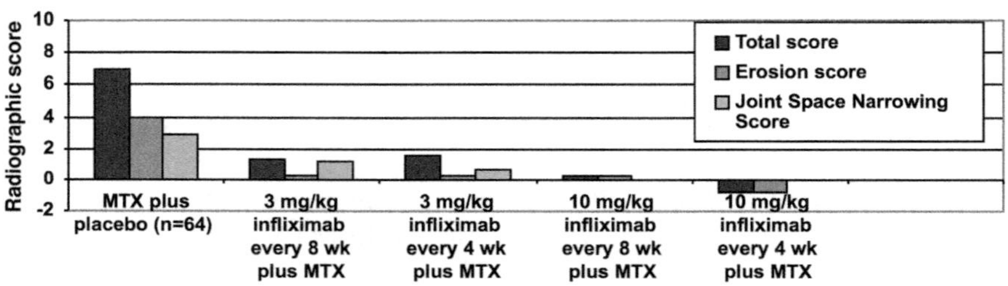

Functional improvement was measured by assessing the change in the HAQ disability index score from baseline through week 102. Infliximab treatment resulted in statistically significant improvement in physical function when compared to placebo. Among the four infliximab treatment groups, HAQ scores were similar. Additionally, using the SF-36 physical component scores, significant improvement was seen in health-related quality-of-life in the patients on infliximab at week 102.

A sub-analysis of ATTRACT data was performed, specifically looking at patients who were ACR20 non-responders to MTX plus infliximab [21]. These patients exhibited mild but statistically significant improvement in Disease Activity Score 28 (DAS28) [22], tender joint count, swollen joint count and CRP level, but did not meet established criteria for ACR20. Analysis showed that radiographic progression in these patients was significantly inhibited compared to ACR20 non-responders to MTX plus placebo (mean change in modified vdH-S score was 6.0 in ACR20 responders, 7.2 in ACR20 non-responders in the MTX plus placebo group *versus* 0.1 in ACR20 responders and 1.2 in ACR20 non-responders in the MTX plus infliximab group).

Building on the concept that very early intervention in rheumatoid arthritis may prevent progression of joint damage, another sub-analysis of ATTRACT data set as its primary objective the evaluation of radiographic damage over 2 years in the early RA cohort of the study [23]. Early RA was defined as fewer than 3 years disease duration. At week 102, erosion and joint space narrowing scores from baseline in the hands and feet decreased significantly in each infliximab dose regimen compared with the MTX plus placebo regimens.

To further evaluate the utility of early, aggressive treatment in RA, ASPIRE (Active-controlled Study of Patients receiving Infliximab for the treatment of Rheumatoid arthritis of Early onset study group) was designed [24]. This study is the largest trial to date of infliximab in patients with RA. 1,049 MTX-naïve patients (up to 3 months of MTX therapy) were randomized to three groups: MTX plus placebo, MTX plus infliximab 3 mg/kg, and MTX plus infliximab 6 mg/kg. Infusions were administered at weeks 0, 2 and 6 and every 8 weeks thereafter through week 46. MTX doses were escalated to 20 mg/week in most patients. Premature discontinuation by patients was similar among the three treatment groups, with more patients withdrawing due to lack of efficacy in the MTX plus placebo group (9.6%) *versus* MTX plus infliximab 3 mg/kg (1.9%) or MTX plus infliximab 6 mg/kg (3.3%). More patients withdrew due to adverse events in the infliximab groups (9.5% in the 3 mg/kg group and 9.6% in the 6 mg/kg group) than MTX plus placebo (3.2%). The primary endpoint for signs and symptoms was the ACR-N (percentage of ACR improvement) from baseline to week 54. Additionally, changes in signs and symptoms were also evaluated using the ACR20 criteria and DAS28 score. Radiographic change was assessed using the change in vdH-S score from baseline to week 54. Physical function was evaluated using the HAQ score averaged over weeks 30–54. Finally, quality of life was estimated using the SF-36.

Patients in the MTX plus infliximab groups achieved a significantly higher median ACR-N than those in the MTX plus placebo groups (38.9% with MTX plus infliximab 3 mg/kg and 46.7% with MTX plus infliximab 6 mg/kg *versus* 26.4% with MTX plus placebo). There were no significant differences in clinical efficacy among the different infliximab dosage groups. Additionally, ACR20, ACR50 and ACR70 response rates were significantly higher in the MTX plus infliximab groups *versus* MTX plus placebo. The ACR90 response rate was significantly higher in the MTX plus infliximab 6 mg/kg group *versus* MTX plus placebo. Greater reductions in DAS28 scores were also observed in the infliximab groups *versus* placebo.

Evaluation of vdH-S score changes from baseline to week 54 favored the MTX plus infliximab group *versus* MTX plus placebo. The mean change in vdH-S was 0.4 ± 5.8 for the MTX plus infliximab 3 mg/kg, 0.5 ± 5.6 for the MTX plus infliximab 6 mg/kg *versus* 3.7 ± 9.6 for the MTX plus placebo group, indicating that patients treated with infliximab had less radiographic progression of disease.

HAQ scores demonstrated greater improvement in the MTX plus infliximab groups than in the MTX plus placebo group. Physical components of the SF-36 also significantly improved in the infliximab treated groups when compared to MTX plus placebo.

The Behandel-Stetegieën (BeSt) trial, a multicenter, single blind, randomized study, compared multiple treatment regimens in patients with early RA, including infliximab plus MTX [25]. These patients (n = 508) had RA for 2 or fewer years without any history of prior DMARD therapy and were randomized to four different groups. Patients in group 1 (n = 125) were placed on sequential monotherapy starting with MTX up to 25 mg/week, followed by sulfasalazine (SSA), then leflunomide. Patients in group 2 (n = 122) were placed on step-up therapy starting with MTX, adding SSA, then hydroxychloroquine (HCQ). Patients in group 3 (n = 133) were placed on step-down therapy starting with MTX + SSA + prednisone 60 mg tapered to 7.5 mg daily. Patients in group 4 (n = 128) underwent treatment with MTX (7.5 mg/wk for 2 weeks, then 15 mg/wk) and infliximab (3 mg/kg at week 0, 2 and 6, then every 8 weeks, doses increased or reduced depending on DAS44). DAS44, HAQ, and vdH-S were measured. The goal of treatment adjustments (allowed at 3 month intervals) was to attain a DAS 44 ≤ 2.4.

Groups 3 and 4 demonstrated a significantly more rapid reduction in HAQ scores at 3 months when compared to groups 1 and 2, though by 1 year, HAQ reductions were similar in all groups. However, median vdH-S score progression was significantly less at 12 months in groups 3 and 4, indicating better radiographic outcomes for these groups.

Quinn et al. confirmed the benefit of treatment with infliximab in very early RA in a 12 month, double-blind, placebo-controlled trial [26]. 20 patients with less than 12 months of symptoms and poor prognostic markers [rheumatoid factor (RF) positivity, possession of the shared epitope, high CRP, female sex and high HAQ score] were enrolled and randomized to placebo or a standard dose of infliximab (3 mg/kg) with escalating doses of MTX for 12 months.

Synovitis measured by magnetic resonance imaging (MRI) was significantly less in the infliximab treated group than in the placebo group by week 14. Additionally, at week 14, the infliximab group demonstrated significantly greater ACR responses than the placebo group (ACR20 was 60% *versus* 20%, ACR50 was 60% *versus* 0%, ACR70 was 60% *versus* 0%). By week 54, no new MRI erosions were noted in the infliximab group, a significantly better response than in the placebo group. At 54 weeks, responder rates began to converge between the MTX plus infliximab and MTX plus placebo groups, with ACR20 responses of 80% and 60%, respectively, ACR50 responses of 80% and 40%, respectively, and ACR70 responses of 70% and 30%, respectively. Importantly, despite withdrawal of infliximab therapy at week 46, functional and quality of life outcomes were sustained in the majority of patients in this group.

Ankylosing spondylitis

The most common subtype of the spondyloarthropathies is ankylosing spondylitis (AS), which primarily manifests with inflammatory back pain and inflammation of the sacroiliac joints [27]. Traditionally, spondyloarthropathy (SpA) patients have been treated using non-steroidal anti-inflammatory drugs (NSAIDs) and physiotherapy with variable efficacy, as well as corticosteroids and DMARDs (such as MTX and SSA), which have limited efficacy. In recent years, numerous studies have demonstrated the utility of infliximab in the treatment of AS.

In 2000, two open pilot trials that studied the efficacy of infliximab in spondyloarthropathy were published. Van den Bosch et al. [28] used infliximab in a group of 21 patients with AS (with peripheral and/or axial disease), psoriatic arthritis (PsA) and undifferentiated SpA. After infliximab infusions at weeks 0, 2, and 6, patients demonstrated significant improvements in all global assessments, tender and swollen joint counts and axial joint function up to day 84. Further, patients with psoriatic arthritis showed marked improvement of Psoriasis Area and Severity Index (PASI) [29].

Another 12 week open pilot study was undertaken to establish potential efficacy of infliximab, specifically in the treatment of active AS [30]. TNF-α messenger RNA and protein had been detected in the inflamed sacroiliac joints of AS patients [31, 32]. These findings, in light of the value of infliximab in the treatment of RA, led researchers to believe that TNF-α blockade might be appropriate for use in AS. 11 patients with 3 months of active AS were treated with 3 infusions of 5 mg/kg infliximab at weeks 0, 2 and 6. Endpoints included improved Bath AS Disease Activity Index (BASDAI) [33], as well as Bath AS Functional Index (BASFAI) [34], Bath AS Metrology Index (BASMI) [35] and the SF-36. Patients demonstrated dramatic clinical improvement in all parameters measured. Median improvement in the BASDAI after 4 weeks was 70% (range 41–94%). At weeks 2 and 4, patients showed over 50% improvement in disease activity, function and pain scores. Interestingly, the positive effect persisted through week 12 in 80% of patients. These results supported the idea that infliximab was useful in treating AS and that the regimen warranted further pursuit.

Adding to the evidence supporting the use of infliximab in AS, several studies demonstrated improvements in the synovium of patients with SpA after treatment with infliximab. They showed a significant reduction in synovial lining layer thickness, vascularity, endothelial activation, and infiltration with neutrophils, macrophages and T cells after 12 weeks of therapy when compared to placebo [36, 37].

Braun et al., who conducted one of the first placebo-controlled trial of infliximab in active AS, randomized 35 patients to 5 mg/kg infliximab and 35 patients to placebo at weeks 0, 2 and 6 [38]. Patients were followed through to week 12. The primary endpoint was 50% improvement at week 12, as measured by the BASDAI. Additional endpoints included the BASFAI, BASMI and SF-36. Radiographic change of the vertebral column, sacroiliac joints and other joints were assessed using the Bath AS Radiology Index (BASRI) [39]. Infliximab was found to be effective in all response criteria. 53% of patients receiving infliximab therapy achieved a 50% improvement in BASDAI at week 12 compared to 9% of patients on placebo. Additionally, this improvement was seen very rapidly, with 41% of infliximab-treated patients achieving 50% BASDAI improvement by week 2. Further, all individual components of the BASDAI were significantly improved in the infliximab group. Other clinical outcomes such as the BASFAI, BASMI and SF-36 physical components showed similar improvement with infliximab therapy.

An open observational 1 year extension study of this trial was subsequently completed [40]. Patients who had tolerated infliximab or placebo in the first 3 months entered the open extension trial in which 5 mg/kg of infliximab was administered every 6 weeks. 54 patients were followed through to week 54, at which time both groups (infliximab/infliximab and placebo/infliximab) demonstrated significant achievement and maintenance of 50% BASDAI improvement (47% and 51%, respectively). Additionally, patient's dosage of anti-inflammatory drugs was reduced 70%. Further, BASFAI, BASMI and SF-36 were significantly improved. Following this, another extension of the study out to 102 weeks was completed [41]. 49 patients were continued on infliximab 5 mg/kg every 6 weeks. At week 102, a significant number of the infliximab/infliximab and placebo/infliximab groups had achieved 50% BASDAI improvement (41% and 49%, respectively). Thus, 58% of all patients achieved the primary efficacy endpoint of at least 50% reduction of the BASDAI score from baseline to week 102. The recently published results of the 3 year (156 week) open label extension of this study [42] continued to demonstrate sustained benefit of the drug with stability of response rates over the 3 years of treatment. This series of studies demonstrated not only the efficacy, but also the durability of response with infliximab therapy.

In 2002, Van den Bosch et al. [43] published results from another randomized double-blind trial comparing infliximab *versus* placebo in 40 patients with active SpA (patients had AS with and without peripheral arthritis, PsA and undifferentiated SpA). Patients were given either placebo or infliximab 5 mg/kg at weeks 0, 2 and 6. The primary endpoints of patient and physician global assessments of disease activity on a visual analog scale at 12 weeks demonstrated significant improvement in the infliximab group over the placebo group. Results were noticeable as early as 2 weeks after first infusion.

While the aforementioned studies did not include patients with significant co-morbidity (including gastrointestinal disease) or allow patients to continue on any DMARD therapy, Generini et al. [44] conducted a small study using infliximab in patients with SpA associated with Crohn's disease. 24 patients with either active or inactive disease were treated with infliximab for 12–18 months. Their control group was another set of SpA/Crohn's patients who were treated with conventional therapy. In this group of patients, infliximab was found to significantly improve not only overall articular symptoms, spinal pain and peripheral arthritis, but also improved gastrointestinal symptoms and prevented inflammatory bowel disease reactivation.

The Ankylosing Spondylitis Study for the Evaluation of Recombinant infliximab Therapy (ASSERT) [45] was a multicenter, placebo-controlled trial that included 279 patients with active AS, randomized to receive 5 mg/kg infliximab or placebo at weeks 0, 2, 6, 12 and 18. Patients were allowed to take concurrent, stable dose of NSAIDs, acetaminophen or tramadol, but were not allowed to take concurrent DMARD or steroid therapy. The primary endpoint of this trial was the achievement of 20% improvement response according to the criteria of the Assessment in Ankylosing Spondylitis (ASAS) International Working Group at week 24 [46]. Infliximab was found to be significantly more effective than placebo in the treatment of AS; ASAS20 response was achieved by 61.2% of the infliximab recipients *versus* 19.2% of placebo patients. Once again, these results were achieved rapidly, with 50% of infliximab treated patients achieving ASAS20 within 2 weeks of beginning infusions. Significantly more patients in the infliximab group achieved ASAS50 criteria. Additionally, BASDAI, BASFAI, BASMI, CRP levels and SF-36 physical component scores significantly improved when compared to placebo.

In December, 2004, the FDA approved infliximab for use in the treatment of ankylosing spondylitis.

Psoriasis and psoriatic arthritis

Psoriasis and psoriatic arthritis (PsA) share immunopathological features, demonstrated on several levels [47]. There is evidence of similar lymphocytic infiltration with CD8+ T cells in both early psoriatic skin lesions and the synovial tissue of PsA, supporting the notion of an HLA Class I driven pathogenesis in both entities. Angiogenesis is a striking feature of early psoriasis and psoriatic arthritis. Elevated levels of vascular endothelial growth factor (VEGF), transforming growth factor-β (TGF-β) and other promoters of angiogenesis are found in synovial fluid of PsA patients. These factors are also co-localized in the peri-vascular regions of both synovial tissue and psoriatic skin lesions. Another common denominator linking psoriasis and PsA is the amplified presence of TNF-α. The role of TNF-α in the pathogenesis of disease is speculated to be several-fold: it has been shown to promote angiogenesis, to upregulate cellular adhesion molecules leading to increased lymphocytic infiltration and to signal keratinocyte hyperproliferation in the skin and protease production in joint cartilage degradation.

Goedkoop et al. assessed the effects of infliximab on both skin and synovial tissues at the cellular level [48]. In this prospective double-blind study, 12 patients with both active PsA and psoriatic skin lesions were randomized to receive a single infusion of either infliximab 3 mg/kg or placebo. At baseline and 48 h after infusion, synovial and skin biopsies were obtained from all patients. At baseline, the inflammatory infiltrate in the tissues of both groups were similar. However, at 48 h, there was a significant decrease in the number of both epidermal and synovial T cells in the infliximab-treated group compared to placebo. Additionally, the infliximab-treated groups demonstrated a significant reduction in the number of macrophages in the synovial sublining.

The strongest evidence of a common pathogenesis in psoriasis and PsA comes from the excellent clinical response derived from TNF-α blockade in treated patients with both joint and skin disease. In a small open label study, Ogilvie et al. demonstrated significant improvement in both psoriatic skin lesions and psoriatic joint disease with infliximab [49]. 6 patients with long-standing, progressive joint and skin disease, despite aggressive DMARD therapy (MTX or SSA) were treated with 5 mg/kg infliximab at weeks 0, 2 and 6 in addition to their previous doses of MTX or SSA. After 10 weeks, patients demonstrated remarkable improvement in PASI score, as well as significant improvement in their arthritis.

In a 30 week multicenter, prospective, open pilot study Salvarani et al. evaluated the safety and efficacy of infliximab in treating resistant psoriatic arthritis [50]. 16 patients with active peripheral arthritis and a history of minimally effective MTX use were treated with 3 mg/kg infliximab, administered at weeks 0, 2, 6, 14, 22 and 30 in addition to their previous MTX regimen. These patients showed significant reductions in multiple disease measures, including swollen and tender joint count, pain, and HAQ starting at week 2 and persisting through to week 30. By week 30, 64% of patients had achieved ACR20 criteria, while 57% of patients satisfied both ACR50 and ACR70 criteria for peripheral joint improvement. Inflammatory measures, such as erythrocyte sedimentation rate (ESR) and CRP were significantly reduced. Psoriasis, as measured by the PASI, improved by 86% at week 30. Of the 3 patients who had axial disease in addition to peripheral joint disease, spinal pain and stiffness was nearly resolved by week 2 – this improvement was sustained through the end of the study.

In April, 2005, results from the largest multicenter, randomized, double-blind, placebo-controlled trial of infliximab in the treatment of PsA were published [51]. The Infliximab Multinational Psoriatic Arthritis Controlled Trial (IMPACT) evaluated 104 patients with PsA who had previously been treated with at least one DMARD without significant clinical efficacy. The initial phase of the trial was blinded, with patients receiving infusions of either 5 mg/kg infliximab (n = 52) or placebo (n = 52) at weeks 0, 2, 6 and 14. For the second phase, placebo patients were started on infliximab therapy, while the infliximab group continued to receive infliximab, now at 8 week intervals. Patients were allowed to receive concomitant therapy with one other DMARD.

The primary endpoint of Phase 1 was the satisfaction of ACR20 criteria at week 16. Infliximab-treated patients achieved a significantly higher proportion of ACR20 responses than the placebo-treated patients (65% and 10%, respectively). 46% and 29% of infliximab-treated patients achieved ACR50 and ACR70 responses, respectively, at week 16. No patient in the placebo group met ACR50 or ACR70 criteria at 16 weeks. After infliximab induction therapy, the placebo group patients demonstrated a pattern of initial clinical response similar to that seen in the infliximab group. By week 50, ACR responses in the two groups were comparable.

PASI scores were also evaluated in this study. Patients with PASI scores ≥2.5 at baseline were included for dermatologic assessment. By week 16, the infliximab group showed a mean improvement of 86% in their PASI score. In contrast, the placebo group demonstrated a 12% worsening of the PASI score. Improved PASI score in the infliximab group was sustained through to week 50. Once the placebo group was initiated on infliximab, their PASI scores dramatically improved; by week 50, their scores were comparable to the infliximab/infliximab group.

Additional measurements, such as individual HAQ components, DAS28, dactylitis and enthesitis scoring, Psoriatic Arthritis Response Criteria (PsARC) [52] and inflammatory measures (ESR, CRP) were also significantly improved in the infliximab group when compared to placebo.

Based on data from IMPACT, in May 2005, the FDA approved the use of infliximab for the treatment of psoriatic arthritis.

Promising reports of infliximab use in rheumatology

TNF-α inhibition has proven beneficial in the treatment of diseases in which TNF-α is central to disease pathogenesis. Case reports also point toward surprising benefits of TNF-α inhibition in disorders not driven by TNF-α, but in which TNF-α plays a role in the inflammatory cascade, leading to organ damage at a certain stage in the disease process. Reflecting this paradigm, in systemic lupus erythematosus (SLE), thought to be a Th2-driven disease, TNF-α has been shown to be involved at several levels in the pathogenesis of this complex autoimmune disorder [53]. Observations suggest that TNF-α may regulate auto-reactive B cells and regulatory T cells [54, 55]. Herrera-Esparza et al. [56] demonstrated increased expression of TNF-α genes in the kidneys of patients with type III and IV lupus nephritis. Aringer et al. proposed that TNF-α is an essential mediator in lupus nephritis [57]. They treated 6 patients with moderately active SLE (4 with nephritis, 3 with arthritis) with 4 doses of 300 mg of infliximab at 0, 2, 6 and 10 weeks. In 52 weeks of follow-up, disease activity, measured by SLE disease activity index (SLEDAI), SLE index score (SIS) and proteinuria, declined during therapy. Despite increases in titers of double stranded DNA (dsDNA) and anticardiolipin antibodies, none of the patients had an increase in disease activity while on infliximab or during the following 52 weeks. These promising results require further exploration, though one may rationalize the use of infliximab in selected SLE patients that have failed traditional therapies.

Interestingly, a multicenter, randomized, double-blind, placebo-controlled trial studying infliximab in patients with primary Sjogren's Syndrome (SS) found no difference between the treatment and placebo groups in terms of secondary endpoints (such as arthritis, salivary flow rate, lacrimation) [58].

Numerous reports in the literature have accumulated, suggesting that infliximab is effective in treating several manifestations of Behçet's disease [59]. These include sight-threatening pan-uveitis, oral and genital ulcerations, gastrointestinal disease, thrombophlebitis, arthritis and neurologic manifestations

[60–64]. In the ophthalmology literature, there are reports of the use of infliximab in treating multiple forms of uveitis, with varying degrees of success. Lindstedt et al. treated 13 patients with site-threatening uveitis [65]. The 6 patients with Behçet's uveitis responded dramatically after the first infusion, while patients with uveitis of other etiologies showed variable responses.

To date, there have been a limited number of case reports and case series regarding the use of infliximab in the treatment of sarcoidosis [66]. In the majority of these patients, infliximab was indicated for corticosteroid toxicity or for failed steroid therapy in a particular organ, designated by one study as the 'index organ' [67]. Clinical response and steroid sparing benefit was reported with use of infliximab for several index organs, such as lungs, skin, parotid glands, kidneys (interstitial nephritis), eyes (uveitis), liver (hepatic sarcoidosis) and CNS (neurosarcoidosis) [68–72].

The systemic vasculidites are a group of rheumatologic disorders that can have organ- and life-threatening consequences. They frequently require heavy immunosuppression with cytotoxic agents and have high risk of complications. Incomplete responses and disease relapse are common. TNF-α participates in the cytokine cascade leading to vascular damage in vasculitis. In this setting, clinical case reports have emerged demonstrating partial or complete success with the use of infliximab in both granulomatous and immune-complex mediated vasculidites. Bartolucci et al. (7 patients) and Lamprecht et al. (6 patients) showed prompt symptomatic response in the majority of patients treated with infliximab for Wegener's, not responsive to conventional treatment [73, 74]. Arbach et al. treated 2 patients with Churg-Strauss syndrome that were refractory to cyclophosphamide and steroids using infliximab with promising results [75]. Limited data suggests that the administration of infliximab may be useful for the treatment of relapsing polymyalgia rheumatica (PMR) and giant cell arteritis (GCA) patients previously treated with steroids [76, 77]. However, a Phase II randomized, controlled study to obtain preliminary evidence of safety and efficacy of infliximab in 44 patients newly diagnosed with GCA (not having failed corticosteroid therapy) was recently conducted. The trial was suspended after an interim analysis at 22 weeks due to a similar proportion of relapse free subjects between the two treatment groups [78]. According to clinical data from an open label trial, it appears that infliximab may be effective when utilized to treat Takayasu's Arteritis [79]. Scattered case reports also support the use of infliximab in treating other vasculidites, such as rheumatoid vasculitis, necrotizing skin vasculitis, with hepatitis C associated mixed cryoglobulinemia and Kawasaki's disease. Controlled trials are warranted to expand our understanding of the role of infliximab in treating vasculitis.

Studies have suggested that TNF-α plays a role in various forms of the idiopathic inflammatory myopathies, including polymyositis (PM) and dermatomyositis (DM). Elevated levels of TNF-α have been demonstrated in patients with PM and DM [80, 81], while patients with PM and DM have had symptomatic improvement with infliximab treatment [82–85].

Anecdotal reports are cited in the literature of infliximab use in rare disorders which lack well-established therapies, such as SAPHO syndrome, Cogan's syndrome, and macrophage activation syndrome/adult Still's disease with varying degrees of success [86]. Although it is unlikely that clinical trials will be conducted for these unusual disorders, TNF-α blockade may be appropriate in individual clinical situations where other options have been exhausted.

Infliximab has proven to be a great addition to the therapies available to the field of rheumatology. Both the basic science research and the clinical experience with infliximab have led to further insights into the pathogenesis of autoimmune disorders. It is a drug that has opened the door to a new way of approaching treatment in rheumatologic disorders by offering a targeted therapeutic regimen, rapid and effective results and an alternative to non-specific immunosuppression.

References

1 Chu CQ, Field M, Feldmann M, Maini RN (1991) Localization of tumor necrosis factor alpha in synovial tissues and at the cartilage-pannus junction in patients with rheumatoid arthritis. *Arthritis Rheum* 34(9): 1125–1132

2 Feldmann M, Brennan FM, Maini RN (1996) Role of cytokines in rheumatoid arthritis. *Annu Rev Immunol* 14: 397–440

3 Williams RO, Feldmann M, Maini RN (1992) Anti-tumor necrosis factor ameliorates joint disease in murine collagen-induced arthritis. *Proc Natl Acad Sci USA* 89(20): 9784–9788

4 Thorbecke GJ, Shah R, Leu CH, Kuruvilla AP, Hardison AM, Palladino MA (1992) Involvement of endogenous tumor necrosis factor alpha and transforming growth factor beta during induction of collagen type II arthritis in mice. *Proc Natl Acad Sci USA* 89(16): 7375–7379

5 Elliott MJ, Maini RN, Feldmann M, Long-Fox A, Charles P, Katsikis P et al (1993) Treatment of rheumatoid arthritis with chimeric monoclonal antibodies to tumor necrosis factor alpha. *Arthritis Rheum* 36(12): 1681–1690

6 Knight DM, Trinh H, Le J, Siegel S, Shealy D, McDonough M et al (1993) Construction and initial characterization of a mouse-human chimeric anti-TNF antibody. *Mol Immunol* 30(16): 1443–1453

7 Harriman G, Harper LK, Schaible TF (1999) Summary of clinical trials in rheumatoid arthritis using infliximab, an anti-TNFalpha treatment. *Ann Rheum Dis* 58 Suppl 1: I61–I64

8 Elliott MJ, Maini RN, Feldmann M, Kalden JR, Antoni C, Smolen JS et al (1994) Randomised double-blind comparison of chimeric monoclonal antibody to tumour necrosis factor alpha (cA2) *versus* placebo in rheumatoid arthritis. *Lancet* 344(8930): 1105–1110

9 Paulus HE, Egger MJ, Ward JR, Williams HJ (1990) Analysis of improvement in individual rheumatoid arthritis patients treated with disease-modifying antirheumatic drugs, based on the findings in patients treated with placebo. The Cooperative Systematic Studies of Rheumatic Diseases Group. *Arthritis Rheum* 33(4): 477–484

10 Kavanaugh AF, Cush JJ, St Clair EW (1996) Anti-TNF-alpha monoclonal antibody (mAb) treatment of rheumatoid arthritis (RA) patients with active disease on methotrexate (MTX); results of a double-blind, placebo controlled multicenter trial. *Arthritis Rheum* 39(suppl): S123

11 Felson DT, Anderson JJ, Boers M, Bombardier C, Furst D, Goldsmith C et al (1995) American College of Rheumatology. Preliminary definition of improvement in rheumatoid arthritis. *Arthritis Rheum* 38(6): 727–735

12 Maini RN, Breedveld FC, Kalden JR, Smolen JS, Davis D, Macfarlane JD et al (1998) Therapeutic efficacy of multiple intravenous infusions of anti-tumor necrosis factor alpha monoclonal antibody combined with low-dose weekly methotrexate in rheumatoid arthritis. *Arthritis Rheum* 41(9): 1552–1563

13 Maini R, St Clair EW, Breedveld F, Furst D, Kalden J, Weisman M et al (1999) Infliximab (chimeric anti-tumour necrosis factor alpha monoclonal antibody) *versus* placebo in rheumatoid

arthritis patients receiving concomitant methotrexate: a randomised phase III trial. ATTRACT Study Group. *Lancet* 354(9194): 1932–1939
14 Lipsky P, van der Heijde DM, St Clair EW, Smolen J, Furst D, Kablen J (2000) 102-week clinical and radiologic results from the ATTRACT trial: a 2 year randomized, controlled, phase 3 trial of infliximab (Remicade) in patients with active RA despite methotrexate. *Arthritis Rheum* 43(Abstract): S269
15 Lipsky PE, van der Heijde DM, St Clair EW, Furst DE, Breedveld FC, Kalden JR et al (2000) Infliximab and methotrexate in the treatment of rheumatoid arthritis. Anti-Tumor Necrosis Factor Trial in Rheumatoid Arthritis with Concomitant Therapy Study Group. *N Engl J Med* 343(22): 1594–1602
16 Maini RN, Breedveld FC, Kalden JR, Smolen JS, Furst D, Weisman MH et al (2004) Sustained improvement over two years in physical function, structural damage, and signs and symptoms among patients with rheumatoid arthritis treated with infliximab and methotrexate. *Arthritis Rheum* 50(4): 1051–1065
17 van der Heijde DM, van Riel PL, Nuver-Zwart IH, Gribnau FW, vad de Putte LB (1989) Effects of hydroxychloroquine and sulphasalazine on progression of joint damage in rheumatoid arthritis. *Lancet* 1(8646): 1036–1038
18 van der Heijde DM (1996) Plain X-rays in rheumatoid arthritis: overview of scoring methods, their reliability and applicability. *Baillieres Clin Rheumatol* 10(3): 435–453
19 Fries JF, Spitz P, Kraines RG, Holman HR (1980) Measurement of patient outcome in arthritis. *Arthritis Rheum* 23(2): 137–145
20 Ware JE, Jr, Sherbourne CD (1992) The MOS 36-item short-form health survey (SF-36). I. Conceptual framework and item selection. *Med Care* 30(6): 473–483
21 Smolen JS, Han C, Bala M, Maini RN, Kalden JR, van der HD et al (2005) Evidence of radiographic benefit of treatment with infliximab plus methotrexate in rheumatoid arthritis patients who had no clinical improvement: a detailed subanalysis of data from the anti-tumor necrosis factor trial in rheumatoid arthritis with concomitant therapy study. *Arthritis Rheum* 52(4): 1020–1030
22 Prevoo ML, 't Hof MA, Kuper HH, van Leeuwen MA, van de Putte LB, van Riel PL (1995) Modified disease activity scores that include twenty-eight-joint counts. Development and validation in a prospective longitudinal study of patients with rheumatoid arthritis. *Arthritis Rheum* 38(1): 44–48
23 Breedveld FC, Emery P, Keystone E, Patel K, Furst DE, Kalden JR et al (2004) Infliximab in active early rheumatoid arthritis. *Ann Rheum Dis* 63(2): 149–155
24 St Clair EW, van der Heijde DM, Smolen JS, Maini RN, Bathon JM, Emery P et al (2004) Combination of infliximab and methotrexate therapy for early rheumatoid arthritis: a randomized, controlled trial. *Arthritis Rheum* 50(11): 3432–3443
25 Goekoop-Ruiterman YP, Vries-Bouwstra JK, Allaart CF, Van Zeben D, Kerstens PJ, Hazes JM et al (2005) Clinical and radiographic outcomes of four different treatment strategies in patients with early rheumatoid arthritis (the BeSt study): A randomized, controlled trial. *Arthritis Rheum* 52(11): 3381–3390
26 Quinn MA, Conaghan PG, O'Connor PJ, Karim Z, Greenstein A, Brown A et al (2005) Very early treatment with infliximab in addition to methotrexate in early, poor-prognosis rheumatoid arthritis reduces magnetic resonance imaging evidence of synovitis and damage, with sustained benefit after infliximab withdrawal: results from a twelve-month randomized, double-blind, placebo-controlled trial. *Arthritis Rheum* 52(1): 27–35
27 Robinson DM, Keating GM (2005) Infliximab: in ankylosing spondylitis. *Drugs* 65(9): 1283–1291
28 Van den BF, Kruithof E, Baeten D, De Keyser F, Mielants H, Veys EM (2000) Effects of a loading dose regimen of three infusions of chimeric monoclonal antibody to tumour necrosis factor alpha (infliximab) in spondyloarthropathy: an open pilot study. *Ann Rheum Dis* 59(6): 428–433
29 Fredriksson T, Pettersson U (1978) Severe psoriasis – oral therapy with a new retinoid. *Dermatologica* 157(4): 238–244
30 Brandt J, Haibel H, Cornely D, Golder W, Gonzalez J, Reddig J et al (2000) Successful treatment of active ankylosing spondylitis with the anti-tumor necrosis factor alpha monoclonal antibody infliximab. *Arthritis Rheum* 43(6): 1346–1352
31 Braun J, Bollow M, Neure L, Seipelt E, Seyrekbasan F, Herbst H et al (1995) Use of immunohistologic and *in situ* hybridization techniques in the examination of sacroiliac joint biopsy specimens from patients with ankylosing spondylitis. *Arthritis Rheum* 38(4): 499–505

32 Braun J, Bollow M, Seyrekbasan F, Haberle HJ, Eggens U, Mertz A et al (1996) Computed tomography guided corticosteroid injection of the sacroiliac joint in patients with spondyloarthropathy with sacroiliitis: clinical outcome and followup by dynamic magnetic resonance imaging. *J Rheumatol* 23(4): 659–664

33 Garrett S, Jenkinson T, Kennedy LG, Whitelock H, Gaisford P, Calin A (1994) A new approach to defining disease status in ankylosing spondylitis: the bath ankylosing spondylitis disease activity index. *J Rheumatol* 21(12): 2286–2291

34 Calin A, Garrett S, Whitelock H, Kennedy LG, O'Hea J, Mallorie P et al (1994) A new approach to defining functional ability in ankylosing spondylitis: the development of the bath ankylosing spondylitis functional index. *J Rheumatol* 21(12): 2281–2285

35 Jenkinson TR, Mallorie PA, Whitelock HC, Kennedy LG, Garrett SL, Calin A (1994) Defining spinal mobility in ankylosing spondylitis (AS). The Bath AS Metrology Index. *J Rheumatol* 21(9): 1694–1698

36 Baeten D, Kruithof E, Van den BF, Demetter P, Van Damme N, Cuvelier C et al (2001) Immunomodulatory effects of anti-tumor necrosis factor alpha therapy on synovium in spondylarthropathy: histologic findings in eight patients from an open-label pilot study. *Arthritis Rheum* 44(1): 186–195

37 Kruithof E, Baeten D, Van den BF, Mielants H, Veys EM, De Keyser F (2005) Histological evidence that infliximab treatment leads to downregulation of inflammation and tissue remodelling of the synovial membrane in spondyloarthropathy. *Ann Rheum Dis* 64(4): 529–536

38 Braun J, Brandt J, Listing J, Zink A, Alten R, Golder W et al (2002) Treatment of active ankylosing spondylitis with infliximab: a randomised controlled multicentre trial. *Lancet* 359(9313): 1187–1193

39 MacKay K, Mack C, Brophy S, Calin A (1998) The Bath Ankylosing Spondylitis Radiology Index (BASRI): a new, validated approach to disease assessment. *Arthritis Rheum* 41(12): 2263–2270

40 Braun J, Brandt J, Listing J, Zink A, Alten R, Burmester G et al (2003) Long-term efficacy and safety of infliximab in the treatment of ankylosing spondylitis: an open, observational, extension study of a three-month, randomized, placebo-controlled trial. *Arthritis Rheum* 48(8): 2224–2233

41 Braun J, Brandt J, Listing J, Zink A, Alten R, Burmester G et al (2005) Two year maintenance of efficacy and safety of infliximab in the treatment of ankylosing spondylitis. *Ann Rheum Dis* 64(2): 229–234

42 Braun J, Baraliakos X, Brandt J, Listing J, Zink A, Alten R et al (2005) Persistent clinical response to the anti-TNF-alpha antibody infliximab in patients with ankylosing spondylitis over 3 years. *Rheumatology (Oxford)* 44(5): 670–676

43 Van den BF, Kruithof E, Baeten D, Herssens A, De Keyser F, Mielants H et al (2002) Randomized double-blind comparison of chimeric monoclonal antibody to tumor necrosis factor alpha (infliximab) *versus* placebo in active spondylarthropathy. *Arthritis Rheum* 46(3): 755–765

44 Generini S, Giacomelli R, Fedi R, Fulminis A, Pignone A, Frieri G et al (2004) Infliximab in spondyloarthropathy associated with Crohn's disease: an open study on the efficacy of inducing and maintaining remission of musculoskeletal and gut manifestations. *Ann Rheum Dis* 63(12): 1664–1669

45 van der HD, Dijkmans B, Geusens P, Sieper J, Dewoody K, Williamson P et al (2005) Efficacy and safety of infliximab in patients with ankylosing spondylitis: results of a randomized, placebo-controlled trial (ASSERT). *Arthritis Rheum* 52(2): 582–591

46 Anderson JJ, Baron G, van der HD, Felson DT, Dougados M (2001) Ankylosing spondylitis assessment group preliminary definition of short-term improvement in ankylosing spondylitis. *Arthritis Rheum* 44(8): 1876–1886

47 Veale DJ, Ritchlin C, FitzGerald O (2005) Immunopathology of psoriasis and psoriatic arthritis. *Ann Rheum Dis* 64 Suppl 2: ii26–ii29

48 Goedkoop AY, Kraan MC, Teunissen MB, Picavet DI, de Rie MA, Bos JD et al (2004) Early effects of tumour necrosis factor alpha blockade on skin and synovial tissue in patients with active psoriasis and psoriatic arthritis. *Ann Rheum Dis* 63(7): 769–773

49 Ogilvie AL, Antoni C, Dechant C, Manger B, Kalden JR, Schuler G et al (2001) Treatment of psoriatic arthritis with antitumour necrosis factor-alpha antibody clears skin lesions of psoriasis resistant to treatment with methotrexate. *Br J Dermatol* 144(3): 587–589

50 Salvarani C, Cantini F, Olivieri I, Macchioni P, Padula A, Niccoli L et al (2003) Efficacy of infliximab in resistant psoriatic arthritis. *Arthritis Rheum* 49(4): 541–545

51 Antoni CE, Kavanaugh A, Kirkham B, Tutuncu Z, Burmester GR, Schneider U et al (2005) Sustained benefits of infliximab therapy for dermatologic and articular manifestations of psoriatic arthritis: results from the infliximab multinational psoriatic arthritis controlled trial (IMPACT). *Arthritis Rheum* 52(4): 1227–1236
52 Clegg DO, Reda DJ, Mejias E, Cannon GW, Weisman MH, Taylor T et al (1996) Comparison of sulfasalazine and placebo in the treatment of psoriatic arthritis. A department of veterans affairs cooperative study. *Arthritis Rheum* 39(12): 2013–2020
53 Davis JC, Jr, (2004) Breaking the ice: Testing tumor necrosis factor alpha blockade in lupus. *Arthritis Rheum* 50(10): 3061–3063
54 Crispin JC, Martinez A, Alcocer-Varela J (2003) Quantification of regulatory T cells in patients with systemic lupus erythematosus. *J Autoimmun* 21(3): 273–276
55 Ueda Y, Yang K, Foster SJ, Kondo M, Kelsoe G (2004) Inflammation controls B lymphopoiesis by regulating chemokine CXCL12 expression. *J Exp Med* 199(1): 47–58
56 Herrera-Esparza R, Barbosa-Cisneros O, Villalobos-Hurtado R, Avalos-Diaz E (1998) Renal expression of IL-6 and TNFalpha genes in lupus nephritis. *Lupus* 7(3): 154–158
57 Aringer M, Graninger WB, Steiner G, Smolen JS (2004) Safety and efficacy of tumor necrosis factor alpha blockade in systemic lupus erythematosus: an open-label study. *Arthritis Rheum* 50(10): 3161–3169
58 Mariette X, Ravaud P, Steinfeld S, Baron G, Goetz J, Hachulla E et al (2004) Inefficacy of infliximab in primary Sjogren's syndrome: results of the randomized, controlled Trial of Remicade in Primary Sjogren's Syndrome (TRIPSS). *Arthritis Rheum* 50(4): 1270–1276
59 Sfikakis PP (2002) Behcet's disease: a new target for anti-tumour necrosis factor treatment. *Ann Rheum Dis* 61 Suppl 2: ii51–ii53
60 Arayssi T, Hamra R, Homeidan F, Uthman I, Awwad ST, Mroue K et al (2005) The efficacy of a single dose of infliximab in the treatment of Behcet's disease uveitis. *Clin Exp Rheumatol* 23(3): 427
61 Haugeberg G, Velken M, Johnsen V (2004) Successful treatment of genital ulcers with infliximab in Behcet's disease. *Ann Rheum Dis* 63(6): 744–745
62 Kram MT, May LD, Goodman S, Molinas S (2003) Behcet's ileocolitis: successful treatment with tumor necrosis factor-alpha antibody (infliximab) therapy: report of a case. *Dis Colon Rectum* 46(1): 118–121
63 Sarwar H, McGrath H, Jr, Espinoza LR (2005) Successful treatment of long-standing neuro-Behcet's disease with infliximab. *J Rheumatol* 32(1): 181–183
64 Tugal-Tutkun I, Mudun A, Urgancioglu M, Kamali S, Kasapoglu E, Inanc M et al (2005) Efficacy of infliximab in the treatment of uveitis that is resistant to treatment with the combination of azathioprine, cyclosporine, and corticosteroids in Behcet's disease: an open-label trial. *Arthritis Rheum* 52(8): 2478–2484
65 Lindstedt EW, Baarsma GS, Kuijpers RW, van Hagen PM (2005) Anti-TNF-alpha therapy for sight threatening uveitis. *Br J Ophthalmol* 89(5): 533–536
66 Baughman RP, Iannuzzi M (2003) Tumour necrosis factor in sarcoidosis and its potential for targeted therapy. *BioDrugs* 17(6): 425–431
67 Baughman RP, Lower EE (2001) Infliximab for refractory sarcoidosis. *Sarcoidosis Vasc Diffuse Lung Dis* 18(1): 70–74
68 Baughman RP, Bradley DA, Lower EE (2005) Infliximab in chronic ocular inflammation. *Int J Clin Pharmacol Ther* 43(1): 7–11
69 Doty JD, Mazur JE, Judson MA (2005) Treatment of sarcoidosis with infliximab. *Chest* 127(3): 1064–1071
70 Heffernan MP, Anadkat MJ (2005) Recalcitrant cutaneous sarcoidosis responding to infliximab. *Arch Dermatol* 141(7): 910–911
71 Mandel L, Wolinsky B, Chalom EC (2005) Treatment of refractory sarcoidal parotid gland swelling in a previously reported unresponsive case. *J Am Dent Assoc* 136(9): 1282–1285
72 Thumfart J, Muller D, Rudolph B, Zimmering M, Querfeld U, Haffner D (2005) Isolated sarcoid granulomatous interstitial nephritis responding to infliximab therapy. *Am J Kidney Dis* 45(2): 411–414
73 Bartolucci P, Ramanoelina J, Cohen P, Mahr A, Godmer P, Le Hello C et al (2002) Efficacy of the anti-TNF-alpha antibody infliximab against refractory systemic vasculitides: an open pilot study on 10 patients. *Rheumatology (Oxford)* 41(10): 1126–1132
74 Lamprecht P, Voswinkel J, Lilienthal T, Nolle B, Heller M, Gross WL et al (2002) Effectiveness

of TNF-alpha blockade with infliximab in refractory Wegener's granulomatosis. *Rheumatology (Oxford)* 41(11): 1303–1307
75 Arbach O, Gross WL, Gause A (2002) Treatment of refractory Churg-Strauss-Syndrome (CSS) by TNF-alpha blockade. *Immunobiology* 206(5): 496–501
76 Cantini F, Niccoli L, Salvarani C, Padula A, Olivieri I (2001) Treatment of longstanding active giant cell arteritis with infliximab: report of four cases. *Arthritis Rheum* 44(12): 2933–2935
77 Salvarani C, Cantini F, Niccoli L, Catanoso MG, Macchioni P, Pulsatelli L et al (2003) Treatment of refractory polymyalgia rheumatica with infliximab: a pilot study. *J Rheumatol* 30(4): 760–763
78 Hoffman GS, Cid MC, Weyand CM, Stone JH, Rendt KE, Salvarani C (2005) Phase II study of the safety and efficacy of infliximab in giant cell arteritis (GCA): 22 week interim analysis. Arthritis Rheum 52(abstract): S271
79 Hoffman GS, Merkel PA, Brasington RD, Lenschow DJ, Liang P (2004) Anti-tumor necrosis factor therapy in patients with difficult to treat Takayasu arteritis. *Arthritis Rheum* 50(7): 2296–2304
80 Kuru S, Inukai A, Liang Y, Doyu M, Takano A, Sobue G (2000) Tumor necrosis factor-alpha expression in muscles of polymyositis and dermatomyositis. *Acta Neuropathol (Berl)* 99(5): 585–588
81 Lundberg I, Ulfgren AK, Nyberg P, Andersson U, Klareskog L (1997) Cytokine production in muscle tissue of patients with idiopathic inflammatory myopathies. *Arthritis Rheum* 40(5): 865–874
82 Anandacoomarasamy A, Howe G, Manolios N (2005) Advanced refractory polymyositis responding to infliximab. *Rheumatology (Oxford)* 44(4): 562–563
83 Hengstman GJ, van den Hoogen FH, van Engelen BG (2004) Treatment of dermatomyositis and polymyositis with anti-tumor necrosis factor-alpha: long-term follow-up. *Eur Neurol* 52(1): 61–63
84 Labioche I, Liozon E, Weschler B, Loustaud-Ratti V, Soria P, Vidal E (2004) Refractory polymyositis responding to infliximab: extended follow-up. *Rheumatology (Oxford)* 43(4): 531–532
85 Uthman I, El Sayad J (2004) Refractory polymyositis responding to infliximab. *Rheumatology (Oxford)* 43(9): 1198–1199
86 Aeberli D, Oertle S, Mauron H, Reichenbach S, Jordi B, Villiger PM (2002) Inhibition of the TNF-pathway: use of infliximab and etanercept as remission-inducing agents in cases of therapy-resistant chronic inflammatory disorders. *Swiss Med Wkly* 132(29–30): 414–422

TNF-alpha Inhibitors
Edited by Jeffrey M. Weinberg and Robin Buchholz

Infliximab in dermatology, gastroenterology, and off-label use

Noah Scheinfeld

Department of Dermatology, St. Luke's-Roosevelt Hospital Center and Beth Israel Medical Center, New York, USA

Introduction

Infliximab is a chimeric IgG 1K monoclonal antibody. Its approximate molecular weight is 149,100 daltons. It is composed of human constant and murine variable regions. Infliximab binds specifically to human TNF-α with an association constant of 10^{10} M^{-1}. Infliximab is produced by using a recombinant cell line cultured by continuous perfusion and is purified by a series of steps that includes measures to inactivate and remove viruses [1].

Biological effects of infliximab

TNF-α induces proinflammatory cytokines that include IL-1 and IL-6. These cytokines enhance leukocyte migration by increasing endothelial layer permeability and expression of adhesion molecules by endothelial cells and leukocytes, activation of neutrophil and eosinophil functional activity, and induction of acute phase and other liver proteins [2]. Infliximab neutralizes the biological activity of TNF-α by binding with high affinity to the soluble and transmembrane forms of TNF-α and inhibits binding of TNF-α with its receptors [3]. A related cytokine that utilizes the same receptors as TNF-α, TNF-beta (lymphotoxin α) is not neutralized by infliximab. It has been found to down-regulate IL-18 but not IL-12 and IL-13 [4]. Chemokines are divided on the basis of the protein structure according to cysteine motifs. The CxC group includes such molecules as interleukin-8 and platelet factor 4; the C C group includes such molecules as eotaxin and monocyte chemoattractant protein-3. The CxC group is usually denoted as 'CXCL' for 'CxC ligand'; the CxC receptor is denoted similarly as 'CXCR'. For the C C group, the chemokine ligands are 'CCL' and receptors are 'CCR'. It upregulates the expression of CXC-chemokine receptor type II and magnifies the proliferative activity of CXC-chemokines in human melanocytes [5]. In Crohn's disease, it decreases levels of IL-10 [6]. Apoptosis of monocytes is not responsible for the therapeutic effects of infliximab. However, some of the therapeutic effects of infliximab may be caused by its ability to downregulate proinflammatory cytokines production by monocytes exposed to bacterial antigens [7].

Crohn's disease

Infliximab was first approved by the Food and Drug Administration (FDA) in 1998 as a treatment of moderately to severely active Crohn's disease. Its initial indication was to reduce the signs and symptoms in patients with Crohn's having an inadequate response to conventional therapies. It was also indicated for the treatment of patients with fistulizing Crohn's disease to reduce the number of draining enterocutaneous fistula(s).

The recommended dose of infliximab for the treatment of severe active Crohn's disease in refractory patients is 5 mg/kg intravenously as a single dose. In patients with Crohn's disease with fistula involvement, an initial dose of 5 mg/kg followed by additional 5 mg/kg doses at weeks 2 and 6 is recommended. This dose is often used in other Crohn's disease patients.

The effects of infliximab on the course of Crohn's disease are complex and probably vary based on the effects on autoantibodies and acute phase reactants. Anti-neutrophil cytoplasmic autoantibodies (ANCA) induce neutrophil activation *in vitro* with release of injurious products that can mediate necrotizing vasculitis *in vivo*. ANCA patterns may identify a Crohn's disease subgroup with a better response to infliximab [8]. It appears that treatment of Crohn's disease is accompanied by changes of acute phase proteins and proteosynthetic markers. The assessment of these laboratory markers may be useful in the management of Crohn's disease patients treated with infliximab [9].

Treatment with infliximab is well tolerated and effective in most children and adolescents with Crohn's disease that is refractory to conventional immunosuppressive therapy [10].

Randomized studies have shown that infliximab is effective for the treatment of Crohn's disease. 169 patients with moderate-to-severe Crohn's disease were enrolled in a 24-week placebo-controlled trial of infliximab. Patients were initially randomized to a single dose of 10 or 20 mg/kg infliximab or placebo to assess dose response [11]. Patients were then retreated with 10 mg/kg infliximab or placebo every 8 or 12 weeks to assess subsequent dosing intervals. The primary endpoint was clinical response at week 2, defined as a decrease in the Crohn's Disease Activity Index score $>$ or $=$ 70 points. At week 2, clinical response occurred in 45% of infliximab-treated patients compared with 27% of patients in the placebo group ($P = 0.023$). Patients appeared to benefit from retreatment with infliximab over 24 weeks, but not all of the results for secondary endpoints were statistically significant.

Another randomized controlled trial assessed the benefits of maintenance infliximab therapy in patients with active Crohn's disease who respond to a single infusion of infliximab in 573 patients with a score of at least 220 on the

Crohn's disease activity index (CDAI) received a 5 mg/kg intravenous infusion of infliximab at week 0 [12]. After assessment of response at week 2, patients were randomly assigned repeat infusions of placebo at weeks 2 and 6 and then every 8 weeks thereafter until week 46 (group I), repeat infusions of 5 mg/kg infliximab at the same timepoints (group II), or 5 mg/kg infliximab at weeks 2 and 6 followed by 10 mg/kg (group III). The prespecified co-primary endpoints were the proportion of patients who responded at week 2 and were in remission (CDAI < 150) at week 30 and the time to loss of response up to week 54 in patients who responded. Analyses of the co-primary endpoints were by intention to treat. 335 (58%) patients responded to a single infusion of infliximab within 2 weeks. At week 30, 23 of 110 (21%) of group I patients were in remission, compared with 44 of 113 (39%) group II ($p = 0.003$) and 50 of 112 (45%) group III ($p = 0.0002$) patients. Thus, patients in groups II and III combined were more likely to sustain clinical remission than patients in group I (odds ratio 2.7, 95% CI 1.6–4.6). Throughout the 54-week trial, the median time to loss of response was 38 weeks (IQR 15 to >54) and more than 54 weeks (21 to >54) for groups II and III, respectively, compared with 19 weeks (10–45) for group I ($p = 0.002$ and $p = 0.0002$, respectively).

In another double-blind, randomized, placebo-controlled trial to evaluate the efficacy of infliximab maintenance therapy in 306 adult patients with Crohn's disease and one or more draining abdominal or perianal fistulas of at least three months' duration. Patients received 5 mg of infliximab per kilogram of body weight intravenously on weeks 0, 2, and 6. A total of 195 patients who had a response at weeks 10 and 14 and 87 patients who had no response were then randomly assigned to receive placebo or 5 mg of infliximab per kilogram every 8 weeks and to be followed to week 54. The primary analysis was the time to the loss of response among patients who had a response at week 14 and underwent randomization. The time to loss of response was significantly longer for patients who received infliximab maintenance therapy than for those who received placebo maintenance (more than 40 weeks *versus* 14 weeks, $P < 0.001$). At week 54, 19% of patients in the placebo maintenance group had a complete absence of draining fistulas, as compared with 36% of patients in the infliximab maintenance group ($P = 0.009$) [13].

Cutaneous manifestations of Crohn's disease

Infliximab is a useful agent in the treatment of the dermatological manifestations of Crohn's disease and the broader category of which a part is inflammatory bowel disease (IBD) [14]. Axillary hidradenitis suppurativa in patients with Crohn's disease has been successfully treated with infliximab [15, 16]. It is useful for ameliorating orofacial [17], refractory perineal Crohn's disease [18] and pyostomatitis vegetans [19]. It is an effective agent in the treatment of co-existent Crohn's disease, pyoderma gangrenosum and psoriasis [20] and in longstanding co-incident Crohn's disease and plaque psoriasis [21]. It can also be used to treat metastatic Crohn's disease in children [22] and adults [23]. It has a role in the treatment of perianal Crohn's disease [24] and severe esophageal Crohn's disease [25]. It can be effective in children with Crohn's disease with dermatologic manifestations that include: pyoderma gangrenosum, orofacial involvement, erythema nodosum, and idiopathic lymphedema resistant to other therapies [26].

Rheumatoid arthritis

Infliximab is also indicated by the FDA for the treatment of rheumatoid arthritis. In November 1999, FDA approved it for use in rheumatoid arthritis with methotrexate in patients who had failed methotrexate therapy alone. In September of 2004, the FDA approved an expanded label for infliximab in combination with methotrexate, as a first line regimen to treat patients with moderate to severe rheumatoid arthritis (RA). The expanded label eliminates the requirement that patients must fail to respond to methotrexate, the current standard of treatment for rheumatoid arthritis, before starting on infliximab.

For the treatment of rheumatoid arthritis infliximab is dosed 3 mg/kg of body weight at 0 weeks, 2 weeks and 6 weeks with a maintenance dose of 3 mg/kg every 8 weeks (6×/year).

Randomized clinical studies have demonstrated the utility of infliximab in treating rheumatoid arthritis. In a study of 1, 49 patients with rheumatoid arthritis patients who had active disease and no prior treatment with methotrexate (MTX) or a TNF-α inhibitor patients were randomly assigned in a 4:5:5 ratio to three treatment groups: MTX-placebo, MTX-3 mg/kg infliximab, and MTX-6 mg/kg infliximab [27]. MTX dosages were rapidly escalated to 20 mg/week, and infliximab or placebo infusions were given at weeks 0, 2, and 6, and every 8 weeks thereafter through to week 46. At week 54, the median percentage of American College of Rheumatology improvement (ACR-N) was higher for the MTX-3 mg/kg infliximab and MTX-6 mg/kg infliximab groups than for the MTX-placebo group (38.9% and 46.7% *versus* 26.4%, respectively; $P < 0.001$ for both comparisons). Patients in the MTX-3 mg/kg infliximab and MTX-6 mg/kg infliximab groups also showed less radiographic progression than those receiving MTX alone (mean ± SD changes in van der Heijde modification of the total Sharp score at week 54: 0.4 ± 5.8 and 0.5 ± 5.6 *versus* 3.7 ± 9.6, respectively; $P < 0.001$ for each comparison). In addition, physical function improved significantly more in the MTX-3 mg/kg infliximab and MTX-6 mg/kg infliximab groups than in the MTX-placebo group. Infliximab therapy was associated with a significantly higher incidence of serious infections, especially pneumonia.

Other studies have shown similar results. In a study of 428 patients were randomly assigned to receive MTX plus placebo or infliximab at a dose of 3 or 10 mg/kg plus MTX for 54 weeks, with an additional year of follow-up [28]. The protocol was later amended to allow for continued treatment during the second year. Of 259 patients who entered the second year of treatment, 216 continued to receive infliximab plus MTX for 102 weeks. 94 of these 259 patients experienced a gap in therapy of >8 weeks before continuing therapy. Infusions were administered at weeks 0, 2, and 6, followed by treatment every 4 weeks or every 8 weeks (alternating with placebo infusions in the interim 4-week visits) at a dose of 3 or 10 mg/kg for a total of 102 weeks (including the gap in therapy). For safety and efficacy assessments, data on the patients who were randomized to receive treatment, irrespective of whether treatment was administered for 102 weeks, were evaluated using all actual observations available. The efficacy measures included the Health Assessment Questionnaire (HAQ) (physical function), Short Form 36 health survey (SF-36) (health-related quality of life), total radiographic scores (structural damage), and the American College of Rheumatology 20% improvement criteria (ACR20) (signs and symptoms). The infliximab plus MTX regimens resulted in significantly greater improvement in HAQ scores ($P <$ or $= 0.006$) and SF-36 physical component summary scores ($P <$ or $= 0.011$) compared with the MTX-only group. There also was stability in the SF-36 mental component summary score among patients who received the infliximab plus MTX regimens. Median changes from baseline to week 102 in the total radiographic score were 4.25 for patients who received the MTX-only regimen and 0.50 for patients who received the infliximab plus MTX regimen. The proportion of patients achieving an ACR20 response at week 102 varied from 40% to 48% for the infliximab plus MTX groups compared with 16% for the MTX-only group.

Ankylosing spondylitis

The third approved indication for infliximab is for the treatment of active ankylosing spondylitis, a painful, progressive inflammatory condition of the spine that can result in fusion of the spinal vertebrae and structural damage to hips and other joints, which can lead to limited function and disability [29, 30]. In June 2003, the European Union gave it the indication to treat ankylosing spondylitis in patients who have severe axial symptoms, elevated serological markers of inflammatory activity and who have responded inadequately to conventional therapy [31]. In December 2004, infliximab received the indication to treat ankylosing spondylitis in the United States.

The approval for AS in the US was based primarily on the 24-week results of the ASSERT (Ankylosing Spondylitis Study for the Evaluation of Recombinant Infliximab Therapy) trial, which demonstrated that AS patients treated with infliximab achieved significant improvement in signs and symptoms associated with their disease, including reduced spinal pain and increased physical function. ASSERT was a randomized Phase III placebo-controlled, double-blind, 33-center trial conducted in North America and Europe. The trial included 279 patients; 201 patients were treated with infliximab, and 78 patients were given placebo infusions. Patients were given infliximab monotherapy 5 mg/kg infusions at weeks 0, 2 and 6, followed by infusions every 6 weeks. Patients were followed through 102 weeks, and further analyses will evaluate structural damage. The primary endpoint of the ASSERT trial was the proportion of patients demonstrating a 20% or greater improvement in signs and symptoms at 24 weeks as measured by Assessment in Ankylosing Spondylitis Response Criteria (ASAS 20). Patients were assessed at baseline and at 24 weeks by standard AS performance scores.

In the infliximab group, 60% of patients achieved ASAS 20 (Assessment in Ankylosing Spondylitis Response Criteria, a composite score that includes spinal pain, inflammation and functionality) compared with 18% of patients in the placebo group ($p < 0.001$). Clinical benefit was observed in patients receiving infliximab as early as week 2 and was maintained over the 24-week study period. In the infliximab group, minimal disease activity (defined as a value of less than 20 on a scale of 0–100 mm in each of the four ASAS response parameters) was achieved in 22% of patients compared with 1% in the placebo group ($p < 0.001$). Patients receiving infliximab also showed significant improvements in individual measurements of disease activity, function and mobility, as well as improvements in chest expansion, and patient global assessment.

The impact of infliximab on the skin affects all aspects of ankylosing spondylitis. Ankylosing spondylitis can be associated with skin diseases that include pitting edema and livedo [32]. Infliximab treatment has been shown to have efficacy in treating lymphedema associated with ankylosing spondylitis [33].

Psoriasis

Infliximab is in development for the treatment of psoriasis, and is currently approved for psoriatic arthritis. Infliximab is currently undergoing Phase III trials for the treatment of moderate-to-severe stable plaque psoriasis. It appears to be the single most effective treatment for stable plaque psoriasis [34]. A large number of studies have noted that infliximab is a promising psoriatic treatment [35–43]. The remissions that it induces can be long lived [44]. It seems to act on the skin soon after it acts on the joints [45]. The median time to response in one study was 4 weeks in infliximab treated psoriatic patients [46].

Firm evidence supports the efficacy of infliximab for the treatment of psoriasis. In a study with 33 subjects, patients with psoriasis received 5 or 10 mg/kg of infliximab or placebo at weeks 0, 2, and 6 of patients with psoriasis, 82% (5 mg/kg-dose group) and 73% (10 mg/kg-dose group) achieved at least a 75% reduction in the Psoriasis Area and Severity Index (PASI) by or before week 10 [47]. In a different study, the mean PASI score improved from 19.04 to 4.91, again an improvement of about 75% [48]. A different study found a 71.3% improvement in PASI score along with an 82.5% mean reduction in inflammation from baseline based on magnetic resonance imaging (MRI) findings [49].

In a large multicenter, double-blind, placebo-controlled trial of infliximab, 249 patients with severe plaque psoriasis were randomly assigned to receive intravenous infusions of either 3 or 5 mg/kg of infliximab or placebo given at weeks 0, 2, and 6. The primary endpoint was the proportion of patients who achieved at least 75% improvement in Psoriasis Area and Severity Index score from baseline at week 10 [50]. At week 26, patients whose Physician Global Assessment indicated moderate or severe disease could receive a single intravenous infusion of their assigned treatment to assess the safety of retreatment after a 20-week, treatment-free interval. At week 10, 72% of patients treated with infliximab (3 mg/kg) and 88% of patients treated with infliximab (5 mg/kg) achieved a 75% or greater improvement from baseline in Psoriasis Area and Severity Index score compared with 6% of patients treated with placebo ($P < .001$). Improvement was observed in both infliximab groups as early as 2 weeks. Overall, 63%, 78%, and 79% of patients in the placebo, 3-, and 5-mg/kg groups, respectively, reported one or more adverse events.

Non-plaque psoriasis is responsive to infliximab. Pustular psoriasis responds rapidly to treatment with infliximab [51] even when severe [52]. It is also useful in treating erythrodermic, recalcitrant psoriasis [53]. It was helpful in treating an HIV positive patient with Reiter's Syndrome [54].

Infliximab can be combined with other medications to treat recalcitrant psoriasis [55]. Reported effective combinations include: infliximab and hydroxyurea [56] and infliximab and methotrexate [57, 58]. Specifically, the combination of methotrexate and infliximab is useful in treating psoriasis and other diseases because it decreases 1) antibodies against infliximab, 2) antinuclear antibody production and 3) development of the 'lupus like syndrome' associated with infliximab.

Psoriatic arthritis

In September 2004, the European Commission gave approval for expanded labeling for infliximab in combination with methotrexate, for the treatment of active and progressive psoriatic arthritis in patients who have responded inadequately to disease modifying anti-rheumatic drugs. It is also approved in the US for this indication. A number of studies have shown that infliximab is effective for the treatment of psoriatic arthritis [59, 60]. It can also be used to good effect in psoriasis resistant to methotrexate [61]. Its utility in the treatment of psoriatic arthritis has been reviewed approvingly by several researchers [62, 63].

A large trial has shown the effectiveness of infliximab in treating psoriatic arthritis [64]. In a Phase III, double-blind trial further researchers evaluated the efficacy of infliximab in active psoriatic arthritis (PsA), as observed in the smaller IMPACT trial. 200 patients with active PsA unresponsive to prior therapy were randomized to infusions of infliximab 5 mg/kg or placebo at weeks 0, 2, 6, 14 and 22. Patients with inadequate response entered early escape at week 16. The primary measure of clinical response was ACR 20. Other measures included Psoriatic Arthritis Response Criteria (PsARC), Psoriasis Area and Severity Index (PASI), and dactylitis and enthesopathy assessments. At week 14, 58.0% of infliximab patients and 11.0% of placebo patients achieved an ACR 20 response and 77% of infliximab patients and 27.0% of placebo patients achieved PsARC (both $p < 0.001$). Among the 85% of patients with at least 3% body surface area psoriasis involvement at baseline, 63.9% of infliximab patients had at least 75% improvement in PASI compared with 2.3% of placebo patients at week 14 ($p < 0.001$). These therapeutic effects were maintained through the last evaluation (week 24). Fewer infliximab patients than placebo patients had dactylitis at week 14 (18.2% *versus* 30.0%; $p = 0.025$) and week 24 (11.8% *versus* 34.0%; $p < 0.001$). Fewer infliximab patients (22.2%) than placebo patients (33.7%) had active enthesopathy at week 14 ($p = 0.016$); corresponding figures at week 24 were 20.4% and 37.2% ($p = 0.002$). Infliximab was generally well tolerated, with a similar incidence of adverse events in each group.

Ulcerative colitis

Centocor, Inc, announced in December 2004 that infliximab has received a Fast Track Designation from the US FDA for the treatment of active ulcerative colitis (UC), a chronic and debilitating disease of the colon, or large intestine, that affects nearly a half million people in the United States. The use of infliximab has been studied and the data less compelling heretofore than for the treatment of Crohn's disease [65, 66]. Kohn studied 13 patients with severe UC, refractory to therapy with methyl-prednisolone, 60 mg IV daily were treated with a single intravenous infusion of infliximab 5 mg/kg [67]. 10 out of 13 patients (77%) had a clinical response to therapy defined by a CAI < or = 10 on two consecutive days. 2 patients (15%) underwent total colectomy because of clinical worsening; one patient refused surgery and was lost to follow-up. Infusion with infliximab produced no significant adverse events. The mean time of follow-up was 25.6 months (range 17–24); in this period of time 8 out of 10 patients (80%) maintained clinical remission and were able to discontinue corticosteroids therapy. Infliximab seems to be as effective as steroids in the management of moderate-to-severe steroid-dependent ulcerative colitis [68].

On September 15, 2005, infliximab was approved by the FDA for reducing signs and symptoms, achieving clinical remission and mucosal healing and eliminating corticosteroid use in patients with moderately to severely active UC who have had an inadequate response to conventional therapy. This approval was based on data published on December 8, 2005, in *The New England Journal of Medicine* that demonstrated the benefits of treatment with infliximab in patients with UC. At week 8, in both the 54-week ACT 1 trial and the 30-week ACT 2 trial, statistically significant differences in the proportion of patients in clinical response, clinical remission, and with mucosal healing were shown in UC patients treated with Remicade *versus* those receiving placebo. On January 30, 2006, the Committee for Medicinal Products for Human Use (CHMP) of the European Medicines Agency (EMEA) issued a positive opinion recommending the approval of an expanded indication of infliximab to include treatment of moderately to severely active UC in patients who have had an inadequate response to conventional therapy, including corticosteroids and 6-mercaptopurine or azothioprine, or who are intolerant to or have medical contraindications for such therapies. Currently, there are no biologic therapies approved to treat moderately to severely active UC in the European Union (EU), hence patients have limited treatment options.

Sarcoidosis

Infliximab is one of the most effective medications at treating all types of sarcoidosis. It is useful in the treatment of sarcoidosis [69, 70], refractory neurosarcoidosis [71], neurosarcoidosis [72], optic neurosarcoidosis [73] and cutaneous sarcoidosis [74, 75]. It is also effective in treating interferon-α-associated sarcoidosis [76]. Isolated sarcoid granulomatous interstitial nephritis responds to infliximab therapy [77].

Hidradenitis suppurativa

Infliximab has the best reports of success of any medication for the treatment of hidradenitis suppurativa. Severe hidradenitis suppurativa without co-morbid conditions is responsive to infliximab [78–80]. Sustained response to infliximab has been found in the SAPHO syndrome, a conditions that manifests with hidradenitis suppurativa [81].

Behcet's disease

Infliximab has been used effectively to treat the manifold manifestations of Behcet's disease [82]. This is even true in severe cases [83] and in children [84]. It has induced remission of this disease [85]. Manifestations of Behcet's disease successfully treated with infliximab include: panuveitis [86], gastrointestinal disease [87], ileocolitis [88], cervical esophageal perforation [89] and recalcitrant orogenital ulceration [90]. It can be used to treat Behcet's disease in cases that have failed to respond to etanercept [91].

Vasculitis

Infliximab can remove the conditions which manifest with vasculitis. It is a useful agent for treating rheumatoid [92] and relapsing vasculitis [93]. It has been used to treat giant cell arteritis [94]; infliximab has been effectively used to treat rheumatoid arthritis-associated vasculitis and cryoglobulinaemia [95]. Infliximab is useful in treating Wegner's granulomatosis [96–98] and Churg-Strauss syndrome [99]. Amyloidosis appears to be a byproduct of inflammation and thus it is not surprising that infliximab can ameliorate amyloidosis. It appears to be a role for infliximab in the treatment of amyloidosis [100]. This is true in both primary and secondary amyloidosis [101].

Graft *versus* host disease

Graft *versus* host disease is a T cell mediated disease that has acute and chronic forms. Both forms have cutaneous manifestations. Because TNF-α is important in the activity of T cells, graft *versus* host disease has been treated with infliximab [102, 103]. In a case of acute graft *versus* host disease with lupus anticoagulant, the lupus anticoagulant disappeared following immunosuppressive therapy with a combination of steroids and infliximab [104]. Infliximab is potentially useful in the treatment of graft *versus* host disease [105, 106] especially in steroid refractory cases [107, 108].

Pyoderma gangrenosum

Infliximab is an effective treatment of pyoderma gangrenosum that occurs either in isolation or in association with systemic disease. In the context of Crohn's disease [109, 110] and inflammatory bowel disease [111], a number of reports have noted its utility in resolving pyoderma gangrenosum and in inducing a remission of this condition [112]. In one study, 8 patients with pyoderma gangrenosum associated with Crohn's disease were treated with infliximab; all had active mucosal inflammation indicated by endoscopic examination, and within 1–4 months, infliximab treatment resulted in complete healing of the pyoderma gangrenosum in three cases (1 parastomal, 2 lower limb), partial healing in three (2 parastomal, 1 lower limb) and temporary improvement in two [113]. Treatment with infliximab leads to the resolution of severe peristomal pyoderma gangrenosum children [114] and adults [115] with peristomal pyoderma gangrenosum.

Uveitis

Infiximab appears to be a promising agent treating autoimmune related uveitis. B27-associated acute anterior uveitis can be treated with it [116]. In treating polyarticular seronegative juvenile idiopathic arthritis, infliximab showed a transient beneficial effect which was more pronounced on uveitis than arthritis [117].

Cutaneous side effects

Infliximab can have a variety of effects on the skin. The most common of these are injections site reactions. In one study a total of 165 consecutive patients who received 479 infliximab infusions acute reactions in 6.1% of cases and delayed reaction in 0.6% of infusions [118]. Another report noted that it caused acute injection site reactions in 3.9% of cases [119]. Another report noted significant infusion reactions have been reported to occur in about 6.9% of patients [120].

A variety of rare side effects have been linked to it as well. A variety of side effects – in particular vasculitis – that paradoxically involve an increase of inflammatory activity have been linked to infliximab. Leukocytoclastic vasculitis [121, 122] and cutaneous vasculitis [123] have been reported secondary to infliximab. Several reports note that it can cause a neuritis [124, 125]. It can induce bullous lesions [126], necrotizing fascitis [127], and cutaneous ulcerations [128]. Crohn's disease treated by infliximab has been associated development of Sweet's syndrome and erythema nodosum [129].

Infliximab can cause 'drug' rashes in the same fashion as other medications. It has caused a drug rash with an interface pattern in four cases [130] and a psoriasiform appearing, lichenoid dermatitis [131]. It can be associated with red man syndrome [132]. In 20 patients treated with infliximab and leflunomide, the commonest adverse event was pruritis associated with an eczematous rash with one case of Stevens-Johnson syndrome [133]. Eczematous drug eruption after infliximab has recently been reported [134]. Infliximab-induced vitiligo has been noted [135]. A niacin-like reaction to infliximab infusion in systemic juvenile rheumatoid arthritis [136]. Infliximab-induced eczematid-like purpura of Doucas and Kapetenakis [137] and an atophic dermatitis like eruption have been induced by infliximab [138]. Its use has been related in adults to the development of nevi [139].

Conclusions

Many skin diseases involve derangement of the immune system, aberrant T cell function and excessive TNF-α production. Thus, it is understandable that infliximab ameliorates many skin diseases. In particular, those diseases that also manifest with arthritis – psoriasis, ankylosing spondylitis, rheumatoid arthritis, ulcerative colitis and Crohn's disease – improve with treatment with infliximab. These diseases and Behcet's disease, pyoderma gangrenosum and hidradentitis supprativa also are accompanied by excessive and aberrant neutrophils, whose function it would seem are normalized with infliximab treatment. The side effects of infliximab include inductions of inflammation (paradoxically), injection site reactions, lymphoma, autoantibodies, lupus and severe infections. These side effects and the substantial cost of infliximab remain barriers to its wide application in dermatology. Nevertheless, because its promise is so great, its indications and uses will undoubtedly expand in the future.

References

1 http://www.rxlist.com/cgi/generic3/infliximab.htm (May 10, 2003)
2 http://www.fda.gov/cber/products/inflcen082498.htm (May 11, 2003)
3 Scallon BJ, Moore MA, Trinh H, Knight DM, Ghrayeb J (1995) Chimeric anti-TNFa monoclonal antibody cA2 binds recombinant transmembrane TNFa and activates immune effector functions. *Cytokine* 7: 251–259
4 Pittoni V, Bombardieri M, Spinelli FR, Scrivo R, Alessandri C, Conti F, Spadaro A, Valesini G (2002) Anti-tumour necrosis factor (TNF) alpha treatment of rheumatoid arthritis (infliximab) selectively down regulates the production of interleukin (IL) 18 but not of IL12 and IL13. *Ann Rheum Dis* 61: 723–725
5 Norgauer J, Dichmann S, Peters F, Mockenhaupt M, Schraufst tter I, Herouy Y (2003) Tumor necrosis factor alpha induces upregulation of CXC-chemokine receptor type II expression and magnifies the proliferative activity of CXC-chemokines in human melanocytes. *Eur J Dermatol* 13: 124–129
6 Detkova Z, Kupcova V, Prikazska M, Turecky L, Weissova S, Jahnova E (2003) Different patterns of serum interleukin 10 response to treatment with anti-tumor necrosis factor alpha antibody (infliximab) in Crohn's disease. *Physiol Res* 52: 95–100
7 Ringheanu M, Daum F, Markowitz J, Levine J, Katz S, Lin X, Silver J (2004) Effects of infliximab on apoptosis and reverse signaling of monocytes from healthy individuals and patients with Crohn's disease. *Inflamm Bowel Dis* 10(6): 801–810
8 Taylor KD, Plevy SE, Yang H, Landers CJ, Barry MJ, Rotter JI, Targan SR (2001) ANCA pattern and LTA haplotype relationship to clinical responses to anti-TNF antibody treatment in Crohn's disease. *Gastroenterology* 120: 1347–1355
9 Kupcova V, Turecky L, Detkova Z, Prikazska M, Keleova A (2003) Changes in acute phase proteins after anti-tumor necrosis factor antibody (infliximab) treatment in patients with Crohn's disease. *Physiol Res* 52: 89–93
10 Lamireau T, Cezard JP, Dabadie A, Goulet O, Lachaux A, Turck D, Maurage C, Morali A, Sokal E, Belli D et al., the French-Speaking Group for Pediatric Gastroenterology Nutrition (2004) Efficacy and tolerance of infliximab in children and adolescents with Crohn's disease. *Inflamm Bowel Dis* 10: 745–750
11 Rutgeerts P, D'Haens G, Targan S, Vasiliauskas E, Hanauer SB, Present DH, Mayer L, Van Hogezand RA, Braakman T, DeWoody KL et al (1999) Efficacy and safety of retreatment with anti-tumor necrosis factor antibody (infliximab) to maintain remission in Crohn's disease. *Gastroenterology* 117: 761–769
12 Hanauer SB, Feagan BG, Lichtenstein GR, Mayer LF, Schreiber S, Colombel JF, Rachmilewitz D, Wolf DC, Olson A, Bao W, Rutgeerts P, ACCENT I Study Group (2002) Maintenance infliximab for Crohn's disease: the ACCENT I randomised trial. *Lancet* 359(9317): 1541–1549
13 Sands BE, Anderson FH, Bernstein CN, Chey WY, Feagan BG, Fedorak RN, Kamm MA, Korzenik JR, Lashner BA, Onken JE et al (2004) Infliximab maintenance therapy for fistulizing Crohn's disease. *N Engl J Med* 350: 876–885
14 Bernstein CN (2002) Treatment of the extraintestinal manifestations of inflammatory bowel disease. *Curr Gastroenterol Rep* 4: 513–516
15 Katsanos KH, Christodoulou DK, Tsianos EV (2002) Axillary hidradenitis suppurativa successfully treated with infliximab in a Crohn's disease patient. *Am J Gastroenterol* 97: 2155–2156
16 Martinez F, Nos P, Benlloch S, Ponce J (2001) Hidradenitis suppurativa and Crohn's disease: response to treatment with infliximab. *Inflamm Bowel Dis* 7: 323–326
17 Mahadevan U, Sandborn WJ (2001) Infliximab for the treatment of orofacial Crohn's disease. *Inflamm Bowel Dis* 7: 38–42
18 Geyer AS, Anhalt GJ, Nousari HC (2000) Effectiveness of infliximab in the treatment of refractory perineal cutaneous Crohn disease. *Arch Dermatol* 136: 459–460
19 Bens G, Laharie D, Beylot-Barry M, Vergier B, Noblesse I, Beylot C, Amouretti M (2003) Successful treatment with infliximab and methotrexate of pyostomatitis vegetans associated with Crohn's disease. *Br J Dermatol* 149: 181–184
20 Tan MH, Gordon M, Lebwohl O, George J, Lebwohl MG (2001) Improvement of Pyoderma gangrenosum and psoriasis associated with Crohn disease with anti-tumor necrosis factor alpha monoclonal antibody. *Arch Dermatol* 137: 930–933
21 Oh CJ, Das KM, Gottlieb AB (2000) Treatment with anti-tumor necrosis factor alpha (TNF-alpha)

monoclonal antibody dramatically decreases the clinical activity of psoriasis lesions. *J Am Acad Dermatol* 42: 829–830
22 de Ridder L, Escher JC, Taminiau JA (2002) Infliximab therapy in children and adolescents with refractory Crohn's disease in the Netherlands; experience with 23 patients. *Ned Tijdschr Geneeskd* 146: 1879–1883
23 Miller AM, Elliott PR, Fink R, Connell W (2001) Rapid response of severe refractory metastatic Crohn's disease to infliximab. *J Gastroenterol Hepatol* 16: 940–942
24 Basu A, Wexner SD (1999) Perianal Crohn's disease. Curr Treat Options. *Gastroenterol* 5: 197–206
25 Heller T, James SP, Drachenberg C, Hernandez C, Darwin PE (1999) Treatment of severe esophageal Crohn's disease with infliximab. *Inflamm Bowel Dis* 5: 279–282
26 Kugathasan S, Miranda A, Nocton J, Drolet BA, Raasch C, Binion DG (2003) Dermatologic manifestations of Crohn disease in children: response to infliximab. *J Pediatr Gastroenterol Nutr* 37: 150–154
27 St Clair EW, van der Heijde DM, Smolen JS, Maini RN, Bathon JM, Emery P, Keystone E, Schiff M, Kalden JR, Wang B et al (2004) Active-controlled study of patients receiving infliximab for the treatment of rheumatoid arthritis of early onset study group. Combination of infliximab and methotrexate therapy for early rheumatoid arthritis: a randomized, controlled trial. *Arthritis Rheum* 50: 3432–3443
28 Maini RN, Breedveld FC, Kalden JR, Smolen JS, Furst D, Weisman MH, St Clair EW, Keenan GF, van der Heijde D, Marsters PA et al (2004) Anti-tumor necrosis factor trial in rheumatoid arthritis with concomitant therapy study group. Sustained improvement over two years in physical function, structural damage, and signs and symptoms among patients with rheumatoid arthritis treated with infliximab and methotrexate. *Arthritis Rheum* 50: 1051–1065
29 Baeten D, Kruithof E, Van den Bosch F, Van den Bossche N, Herssens A, Mielants H, De Keyser F, Veys EM (2003) Systematic safety follow up in a cohort of 107 patients with spondyloarthropathy treated with infliximab: a new perspective on the role of host defence in the pathogenesis of the disease? *Ann Rheum Dis* 62: 829–834
30 Sieper J, Braun J (2001) New treatment options in ankylosing spondylitis: a role for anti-TNFalpha therapy. *Ann Rheum Dis* 60 Suppl 3: 58–61
31 http://www.spondylitis.org/News/NewsDefault.aspx?NewsID=176 (28 January 2004)
32 Marquart-Elbaz C, Lipsker D, Sibilia J, Faivre M, Grosshans E, Cribier B (2002) Painful edema of the feet revealing ankylosing spondylitis. *Ann Dermatol Venereol* 129: 889–891
33 Almodovar R, Zarco P, Quiros FJ, Mazzucchelli R (2004) Infliximab treatment efficacy in lymphoedema associated with ankylosing spondylitis. *Rheumatology (Oxford)* 43: 1456
34 Gottlieb AB, Chaudhari U, Mulcahy LD, Li S, Dooley LT, Baker DG (2003) Infliximab monotherapy provides rapid and sustained benefit for plaque-type psoriasis. *J Am Acad Dermatol* 48: 829–835
35 Schopf RE, Aust H, Knop J (2002) Treatment of psoriasis with the chimeric monoclonal antibody against tumor necrosis factor alpha, infliximab. *J Am Acad Dermatol* 46: 886–891
36 Amital H, Ingber A, Rubinow A (2003) Infliximab-induced remission of extensive plaque psoriasis. *Isr Med Assoc J* 5: 827–828
37 Al-Salem IH (2003) Striking and rapid improvement of plaque psoriasis with infliximab. A report of two cases. *Dermatology* 207: 54–56
38 Gottlieb AB (2003) Infliximab for psoriasis. *J Am Acad Dermatol* 49(2 Suppl): S112–S117
39 Cather JC, Cather JC, Abramovits W (2003) Investigational therapies for psoriasis. *J Am Acad Dermatol* 49(2 Suppl): S133–S138
40 Cather JC, Cather JC, Abramovits W (2003) Investigational therapies for psoriasis. *J Am Acad Dermatol* 49(2 Suppl): S133–S138
41 Mang R, Stege H, Ruzicka T, Krutmann J (2002) Response of severe psoriasis to infliximab. *Dermatology* 204: 156–157
42 O'Quinn RP, Miller JL (2002) The effectiveness of tumor necrosis factor alpha antibody (infliximab) in treating recalcitrant psoriasis: a report of 2 cases. *Arch Dermatol* 138: 644–648
43 Chan JJ, Gebauer K (2003) Treatment of severe recalcitrant plaque psoriasis with single-dose intravenous tumour necrosis factor-alpha antibody (infliximab). *Australas J Dermatol* 44: 116–120
44 Gottlieb AB (2003) Clinical research helps elucidate the role of tumor necrosis factor-alpha in the pathogenesis of T1-mediated immune disorders: use of targeted immunotherapeutics as pathogenic probes. *Lupus* 12: 190–194
45 Wollina U, Konrad H (2002) Treatment of recalcitrant psoriatic arthritis with anti-tumor necrosis

factor-alpha antibody. *J Eur Acad Dermatol Venereol* 16: 127–129
46 Chaudhari U, Romano P, Mulcahy LD, Dooley LT, Baker DG, Gottlieb AB (2001) Efficacy and safety of infliximab monotherapy for plaque-type psoriasis: a randomised trial. *Lancet* 357: 1842–1847
47 Gottlieb AB, Masud S, Ramamurthi R, Abdulghani A, Romano P, Chaudhari U, Dooley LT, Fasanmade AA, Wagner CL (2003) Pharmacodynamic and pharmacokinetic response to anti-tumor necrosis factor-alpha monoclonal antibody (infliximab) treatment of moderate to severe psoriasis vulgaris. *J Am Acad Dermatol* 48: 68–75
48 Cauza E, Spak M, Cauza K, Hanusch-Enserer U, Dunky A, Wagner E (2002) Treatment of psoriatic arthritis and psoriasis vulgaris with the tumor necrosis factor inhibitor infliximab. *Rheumatol Int* 22: 227–232
49 Antoni C, Dechant C, Hanns-Martin Lorenz PD, Wendler J, Ogilvie A, Lueftl M, Kalden-Nemeth D, Kalden JR, Manger B (2002) Open-label study of infliximab treatment for psoriatic arthritis: clinical and magnetic resonance imaging measurements of reduction of inflammation. *Arthritis Rheum* 47: 506–512
50 Gottlieb AB, Evans R, Li S, Dooley LT, Guzzo CA, Baker D, Bala M, Marano CW, Menter A (2004) Infliximab induction therapy for patients with severe plaque-type psoriasis: a randomized, double-blind, placebo-controlled trial. *J Am Acad Dermatol* 51: 534–542
51 Newland MR, Weinstein A, Kerdel F (2002) Rapid response to infliximab in severe pustular psoriasis, von Zumbusch type. *Int J Dermatol* 41: 449–452
52 Elewski BE (2002) Infliximab for the treatment of severe pustular psoriasis. *J Am Acad Dermatol* 47: 796–797
53 Rongioletti F, Borenstein M, Kirsner R, Kerdel F (2003) Erythrodermic, recalcitrant psoriasis: clinical resolution with infliximab. J *Dermatolog Treat* 14: 222–225
54 Gaylis N (2003) Infliximab in the Treatment of an HIV Positive Patient with Reiter's Syndrome. *J Rheumatol* 30: 407–411
55 Lebwohl M (2003) Combining the new biologic agents with our current psoriasis armamentarium. *J Am Acad Dermatol* 49(2 Suppl): S118–S124
56 Gach JE, Berth-Jones J (2003) Successful treatment of recalcitrant psoriasis with a combination of infliximab and hydroxyurea. *J Dermatolog Treat* 14: 226–228
57 Dalaker M, Bonesronning JH (2003) Treatment of severe psoriasis with anti-TNF-alpha-antibody and methotrexate. *Tidsskr Nor Laegeforen* 123: 1070–1071
58 Kirby B, Marsland AM, Carmichael AJ, Griffiths CE (2001) Successful treatment of severe recalcitrant psoriasis with combination infliximab and methotrexate. *Clin Exp Dermatol* 26: 27–29
59 Girolomoni G, Abeni D (2001) Anti-tumor necrosis factor alpha therapy in psoriatic arthritis and psoriasis. *Arch Dermatol* 137: 784–785
60 Antoni C, Manger B (2002) Infliximab for psoriasis and psoriatic arthritis. *Clin Exp Rheumatol* 20: S122–S125
61 Ogilvie AL, Antoni C, Dechant C, Manger B, Kalden JR, Schuler G, Luftl M (2001) Treatment of psoriatic arthritis with antitumour necrosis factor-alpha antibody clears skin lesions of psoriasis resistant to treatment with methotrexate. *Br J Dermatol* 144: 587–589
62 Cassano N, Loconsole F, Amoruso A, Coviello C, Filieri M, Filotico R, Del Vecchio S, Vena GA (2004) Infliximab monotherapy for refractory psoriasis: preliminary results. *Int J Immunopathol Pharmacol* 17: 373–380
63 Yazdani-Biuki B, Wohlfahrt K, Mulabecirovic A, Mueller T, Hermann J, Graninger WB, Brezinschek HP, Brezinschek RI (2004) Long term treatment of psoriatic arthritis with infliximab. *Ann Rheum Dis* 63: 1531–1532; author reply 1532
64 Antoni C, Krueger GG, de Vlam K, Birbara C, Beutler A, Guzzo C, Zhou B, Dooley LT, Kavanaugh A (2005) Infliximab improves signs and symptoms of psoriatic arthritis: results of the IMPACT 2 trial. *Ann Rheum Dis* 64: 1150–1157
65 Ochsenkuhn T, Sackmann M, Goke B (2004) Infliximab for acute, not steroid-refractory ulcerative colitis: a randomized pilot study. *Eur J Gastroenterol Hepatol* 16: 1167–1171
66 Shen EH, Das KM (2004) Current therapeutic recommendations: infliximab for ulcerative colitis. *J Clin Gastroenterol* 38: 741–745
67 Kohn A, Prantera C, Pera A, Cosintino R, Sostegni R, Daperno M (2004) Infliximab in the treatment of severe ulcerative colitis: a follow-up study. *Eur Rev Med Pharmacol Sci* 8: 235–237
68 Armuzzi A, De Pascalis B, Lupascu A, Fedeli P, Leo D, Mentella MC, Vincenti F, Melina D, Gasbarrini G, Pola P, Gasbarrini A (2004) Infliximab in the treatment of steroid-dependent ulcer-

ative colitis. *Eur Rev Med Pharmacol Sci* 8: 231–233
69 Serio RN (2003) Infliximab treatment of sarcoidosis. *Ann Pharmacother* 37: 577–581
70 Ulbricht KU, Stoll M, Bierwirth J, Witte T, Schmidt RE (2003) Successful tumor necrosis factor alpha blockade treatment in therapy-resistant sarcoidosis. *Arthritis Rheum* 48: 3542–3543
71 Morcos Z (2003) Refractory neurosarcoidosis responding to infliximab. *Neurology* 60: 1220–1221
72 Pettersen JA, Zochodne DW, Bell RB, Martin L, Hill MD (2002) Refractory neurosarcoidosis responding to infliximab. *Neurology* 59: 1660–1661
73 Katz JM, Bruno MK, Winterkorn JM, Nealon N (2003) The pathogenesis and treatment of optic disc swelling in neurosarcoidosis: a unique therapeutic response to infliximab. *Arch Neurol* 60: 426–430
74 Mallbris L, Ljungberg A, Hedblad MA, Larsson P, Stahle-Backdahl M (2003) Progressive cutaneous sarcoidosis responding to anti-tumor necrosis factor-alpha therapy. *J Am Acad Dermatol* 48: 290–293
75 Meyerle JH, Shorr A (2003) The use of infliximab in cutaneous sarcoidosis. *J Drugs Dermatol* 2: 413–414
76 Menon Y, Cucurull E, Reisin E, Espinoza LR (2004) Interferon-alpha-associated sarcoidosis responsive to infliximab therapy. *Am J Med Sci* 328: 173–175
77 Thumfart J, Muller D, Rudolph B, Zimmering M, Querfeld U, Haffner D (2005) Isolated sarcoid granulomatous interstitial nephritis responding to infliximab therapy. *Am J Kidney Dis* 45: 411–414
78 Adams DR, Gordon KB, Devenyi AG, Ioffreda MD (2003) Severe hidradenitis suppurativa treated with infliximab infusion. *Arch Dermatol* 139: 1540–1542
79 Lebwohl B, Sapadin AN (2003) Infliximab for the treatment of hidradenitis suppurativa. *J Am Acad Dermatol* 49(5 Suppl): S275–S276
80 Sullivan TP, Welsh E, Kerdel FA, Burdick AE, Kirsner RS (2003) Infliximab for hidradenitis suppurativa. *Br J Dermatol* 149(5): 1046–1049
81 Wagner AD, Andresen J, Jendro MC, Hulsemann JL, Zeidler H (2002) Sustained response to tumor necrosis factor alpha-blocking agents in two patients with SAPHO syndrome. *Arthritis Rheum* 46: 1965–1968
82 Sfikakis PP (2002) Behcet's disease: a new target for anti-tumour necrosis factor treatment. *Ann Rheum Dis* 61 Suppl 2: 51–53
83 Andreu M, Ramanoelina J, Fajnkuchen F, Mouthon L, Cohen P, Laroche L, Guillevin L (2002) Treatment of severe Behcet's disease with anti-TNF-alpha: infliximab. A case report. *Ann Med Interne (Paris)* 153: 414–415
84 Saulsbury FT, Mann JA (2003) Treatment with infliximab for a child with Behcet's disease. *Arthritis Rheum* 49: 599–600
85 Rozenbaum M, Rosner I, Portnoy E (2002) Remission of Behcet's syndrome with TNFalpha blocking treatment. *Ann Rheum Dis* 61: 283–284
86 Sfikakis PP, Theodossiadis PG, Katsiari CG, Kaklamanis P, Markomichelakis NN (2001) Effect of infliximab on sight-threatening panuveitis in Behcet's disease. *Lancet* 358: 295–296
87 Hassard PV, Binder SW, Nelson V, Vasiliauskas EA (2001) Anti-tumor necrosis factor monoclonal antibody therapy for gastrointestinal Behcet's disease: a case report. *Gastroenterology* 120: 995–999
88 Kram MT, May LD, Goodman S, Molinas S (2003) Behcet's ileocolitis: successful treatment with tumor necrosis factor-alpha antibody (infliximab) therapy: report of a case. *Dis Colon Rectum* 46: 118–121
89 Mussack T, Landauer N, Ladurner R, Schiemann U, Goetzberger M, Burchardi C, Folwaczny C, Heldwein W, Hallfeldt K (2003) Successful treatment of cervical esophageal perforation in Behcet's disease with drainage operation and infliximab. *Am J Gastroenterol* 98: 703–704
90 Robertson LP, Hickling P (2001) Treatment of recalcitrant orogenital ulceration of Behcet's syndrome with infliximab. *Rheumatology (Oxford)* 40: 473–474
91 Estrach C, Mpofu S, Moots RJ (2002) Behcet's syndrome: response to infliximab after failure of etanercept. *Rheumatology (Oxford)* 41: 1213–1214
92 Unger L, Kayser M, Nusslein HG (2003) Successful treatment of severe rheumatoid vasculitis by infliximab. *Ann Rheum Dis* 62: 587–588
93 Booth AD, Jefferson HJ, Ayliffe W, Andrews PA, Jayne DR (2002) Safety and efficacy of TNFalpha blockade in relapsing vasculitis. *Ann Rheum Dis* 61: 559

94 Airo P, Antonioli CM, Vianelli M, Toniati P (2002) Anti-tumour necrosis factor treatment with infliximab in a case of giant cell arteritis resistant to steroid and immunosuppressive drugs. *Rheumatology (Oxford)* 41: 347–349
95 Bartolucci P, Ramanoelina J, Cohen P, Mahr A, Godmer P, Le Hello C, Guillevin L (2002) Efficacy of the anti-TNF-alpha antibody infliximab against refractory systemic vasculitides: an open pilot study on 10 patients. *Rheumatology (Oxford)* 41: 1126–1132
96 Lamprecht P, Voswinkel J, Lilienthal T, Nolle B, Heller M, Gross WL, Gause A (2002) Effectiveness of TNF-alpha blockade with infliximab in refractory Wegener's granulomatosis. *Rheumatology (Oxford)* 41: 1303–1307
97 (2002) Induction of remission with infliximab in therapy-refractory Wegener's granulomatosis – Follow-up of six patients. *Dtsch Med Wochenschr* 127: 2346
98 Lam precht P, Arbach O, Voswinkel J, Lilienthal T, Nolle B, Heller M, Gause A, Gross WL (2002) Induction of remission with infliximab in therapy-refractory Wegener's granulomatosis – Follow-up of six patients. *Dtsch Med Wochenschr* 127: 1876–1880
99 Hellmich B, Gross WL (2004) Recent progress in the pharmacotherapy of Churg-Strauss syndrome. *Expert Opin Pharmacother* 5: 25–35
100 Ortiz-Santamaria V, Valls-Roc M, Sanmarti M, Olive A (2003) Anti-TNF treatment in secondary amyloidosis. *Rheumatology (Oxford)* 42: 1425–1426
101 Rysava R, Merta M, Spicka I, Tesar V (2003) Current therapeutic possibilities in primary and secondary amyloidosis and our experience with 31 patients. *Nephrol Dial Transplant* 18 Suppl 5: v38–40
102 Bruner RJ, Farag SS (2003) Monoclonal antibodies for the prevention and treatment of graft-*versus*-host disease. *Semin Oncol* 30: 509–519
103 Kobbe G, Schneider P, Rohr U, Fenk R, Neumann F, Aivado M, Dietze L, Kronenwett R, Hunerliturkoglu A, Haas R (2001) Treatment of severe steroid refractory acute graft-*versus*-host disease with infliximab, a chimeric human/mouse antiTNFalpha antibody. *Bone Marrow Transplant* 28: 47–49
104 Kharfan-Dabaja MA, Morgensztern D, Santos E, Goodman M, Fernandez HF (2003) Acute graft-*versus*-host disease (aGVHD) presenting with an acquired lupus anticoagulant. *Bone Marrow Transplant* 31: 129–131
105 Jacobsohn DA (2002) Novel therapeutics for the treatment of graft-*versus*-host disease. *Expert Opin Investig Drugs* 11: 1271–1280
106 Jacobsohn DA (2003) Emerging therapies for graft-*versus*-host disease. *Expert Opin Emerg Drugs* 8: 323–338
107 Carpenter PA, Sanders JE (2003) Steroid-refractory graft-*versus*-host disease: past, present and future. *Pediatr Transplant* 7 (3 Suppl): 19–31
108 Jacobsohn DA, Hallick J, Anders V, McMillan S, Morris L, Vogelsang GB (2003) Infliximab for steroid-refractory acute GVHD: a case series. *Am J Hematol* 74: 119–124
109 Zaccagna A, Bertone A, Puiatti P, Picciotto F, Sprujevnik T, Santucci R, Rossini FP (2003) Anti-tumor necrosis factor alpha monoclonal antibody (infliximab) for the treatment of Pyoderma gangrenosum associated with Crohn's disease. *Eur J Dermatol* 13: 258–260
110 Triantafillidis JK, Cheracakis P, Sklavaina M, Apostolopoulou K (2002) Favorable response to infliximab treatment in a patient with active Crohn disease and pyoderma gangrenosum. *Scand J Gastroenterol* 37: 863–865
111 Regueiro M, Valentine J, Plevy S, Fleisher MR, Lichtenstein GR (2003) Infliximab for treatment of pyoderma gangrenosum associated with inflammatory bowel disease. *Am J Gastroenterol* 98: 1821–1826
112 Romero-Gomez M, Sanchez-Munoz D (2002) Infliximab induces remission of pyoderma gangrenosum. *Eur J Gastroenterol Hepatol* 14: 907
113 Ljung T, Staun M, Grove O, Fausa O, Vatn MH, Hellstrom PM (2002) Pyoderma gangrenosum associated with crohn disease: effect of TNF-alpha blockade with infliximab. *Scand J Gastroenterol* 37: 1108–1110
114 Batres LA, Mamula P, Baldassano RN (2002) Resolution of severe peristomal pyoderma gangrenosum with infliximab in a child with Crohn disease. *J Pediatr Gastroenterol Nutr* 34: 558–560
115 Mimouni D, Anhalt GJ, Kouba DJ, Nousari HC (2003) Infliximab for peristomal pyoderma gangrenosum. *Br J Dermatol* 148: 813–816
116 El-Shabrawi Y, Hermann J (2002) Anti-tumor necrosis factor-alpha therapy with infliximab as an alternative to corticosteroids in the treatment of human leukocyte antigen B27-associated acute

anterior uveitis. *Ophthalmology* 109: 2342–2346
117 Mangge H, Heinzl B, Grubbauer HM, El-Shabrawi Y, Schauenstein K (2003) Therapeutic experience with infliximab in a patient with polyarticular juvenile idiopathic arthritis and uveitis. *Rheumatol Int* 23: 258–261
118 Cheifetz A, Smedley M, Martin S, Reiter M, Leone G, Mayer L, Plevy S (2003) The incidence and management of infusion reactions to infliximab: a large center experience. *Am J Gastroenterol* 98: 1315–1324
119 Colombel JF, Loftus EV Jr, Tremaine WJ, Egan LJ, Harmsen WS, Schleck CD, Zinsmeister AR, Sandborn WJ (2004) The safety profile of infliximab in patients with Crohn's disease: the Mayo clinic experience in 500 patients. *Gastroenterology* 126: 19–31
120 Farrell RJ, Shah SA, Lodhavia PJ, Alsahli M, Falchuk KR, Michetti P, Peppercorn MA (2000) Clinical experience with infliximab therapy in 100 patients with Crohn's disease. *Am J Gastroenterol* 95: 3490–3497
121 McIlwain L, Carter JD, Bin-Sagheer S, Vasey FB, Nord J (2003) Hypersensitivity vasculitis with leukocytoclastic vasculitis secondary to infliximab. *J Clin Gastroenterol* 36: 411–413
122 McIlwain L, Carter JD, Bin-Sagheer S, Vasey FB, Nord J (2003) Hypersensitivity vasculitis with leukocytoclastic vasculitis secondary to infliximab. *J Clin Gastroenterol* 36: 411–413
123 McCain ME, Quinet RJ, Davis WE (2002) Etanercept and infliximab associated with cutaneous vasculitis. *Rheumatology (Oxford)* 41: 116–117
124 Foroozan R, Buono LM, Sergott RC, Savino PJ (2002) Retrobulbar optic neuritis associated with infliximab. *Arch Ophthalmol* 120: 985–987
125 en Tusscher MP, Jacobs PJ, Busch MJ, de Graaf L, Diemont WL (2003) Bilateral anterior toxic optic neuropathy and the use of infliximab. *BMJ* 326: 579
126 Kent PD, Davis JM 3rd, Davis MD, Matteson EL (2002) Bullous skin lesions following infliximab infusion in a patient with rheumatoid arthritis. *Arthritis Rheum* 46: 2257–2258
127 Chan AT, Cleeve V, Daymond TJ (2002) Necrotising fasciitis in a patient receiving infliximab for rheumatoid arthritis. *Postgrad Med J* 78: 47–48
128 (2003) Cutaneous ulceration with methotrexate. *Prescrire Int* 12: 59–60
129 Vanbiervliet G, Anty R, Schneider S, Arab K, Rampal P, Hebuterne X (2002) Sweet's syndrome and erythema nodosum associated with Crohn's disease treated by infliximab. *Gastroenterol Clin Biol* 26: 295–297
130 Vergara G, Silvestre JF, Betlloch I, Vela P, Albares MP, Pascual JC (2002) Cutaneous drug eruption to infliximab: report of 4 cases with an interface dermatitis pattern. *Arch Dermatol* 138: 1258–1259
131 Verea MM, Del Pozo J, Yebra-Pimentel MT, Porta A, Fonseca E (2004) Psoriasiform eruption induced by infliximab. *Ann Pharmacother* 38: 54–57
132 Lobel EZ, Korelitz BI, Warman JI (2003) Red man syndrome and infliximab. *J Clin Gastroenterol* 36: 186
133 Kiely PD, Johnson DM (2002) Infliximab and leflunomide combination therapy in rheumatoid arthritis: an open-label study. *Rheumatology (Oxford)* 41: 631–637
134 Dumont-Berset M, Laffitte E, Gerber C, Dudler J, Panizzon RG (2004) Eczematous drug eruption after infliximab. *Br J Dermatol* 151: 1272–1273
135 Ramirez-Hernandez M, Marras C, Martinez-Escribano JA (2005) Infliximab-induced vitiligo. *Dermatology* 210: 79–80
136 Becker M, Rose CD, McIlvain-Simpson G (2004) Niacin-like reaction to infliximab infusion in systemic juvenile rheumatoid arthritis. *J Rheumatol* 31: 2529–2530
137 Wang LC, Medenica MM, Shea CR, Busbey S (2003) Infliximab-induced eczematid-like purpura of Doucas and Kapetenakis. *J Am Acad Dermatol* 49: 157–158
138 Wright RC (2003) Atopic dermatitis-like eruption precipitated by infliximab. *J Am Acad Dermatol* 49: 160–161
139 Katsanos KH, Christodoulou DK, Zioga A, Tsianos EV (2003) Cutaneous nevi pigmentosus during infliximab therapy in a patient with Crohn's disease: fallacy or coincidence? *Inflamm Bowel Dis* 9: 279

TNF-alpha Inhibitors
Edited by Jeffrey M. Weinberg and Robin Buchholz

Adalimumab in rheumatology

Harry D. Fischer

Chief Rheumatology, Beth Israel Medical Center, New York, USA

Adalimumab (Humira; Abbott Laboratories, Parsippany, NJ, USA) is a fully humanized anti-TNF-α monoclonal antibody. It is currently approved for use in the treatment of rheumatoid arthritis. Rheumatoid arthritis is a chronic inflammatory disease, which can result in joint destruction and deformity. Although the etiology is unknown it is presumed to be an autoimmune disease. About 0.8% of adults are affected by this disorder [1]. Irreversible joint damage as demonstrated by radiographic changes has been showed to occur early on in the disease process [2]. Current strategies for the treatment of rheumatoid arthritis call for early institution of disease-modifying antirheumatic drugs (DMARDS) often in combination [3].

Previous therapies for rheumatoid arthritis have often been non-specific in their immunosuppressive effects. The introduction of anti-TNF therapy for this disease can be considered a much more selective therapeutic approach. The TNF antagonists, of which adaliuimab is the most recently introduced, are often a very effective treatment. The onset of the therapeutic response is often very rapid [4].

TNF-α has been shown to promote inflammation both directly and through induction of other cytokines. Patients with rheumatoid arthritis have been found to increase levels of TNF-α in both their serum and synovial fluid [5]. These increased levels of TNF-α have been shown to play a major role in the inflammation found in the rheumatoid joint [6].

When drugs are studied for effectiveness in the treatment of rheumatoid arthritis outcome measures established by the American College of Rheumatology (ACR) are often used.

Achieving an ACR 20 requires a 20% reduction in tender and swollen joints. Additionally there must be a 20% reduction in three of five other measures: pain, global assessment of patients and physician, self-assessment of physical disability, and levels of acute phase reactants. Even more important than the ACR 20 is the ACR 50, which requires a 50% improvent in the above parameters. And finally the most important parameter is the ACR 70, which necessitates a 70% improvement in the measures [4].

Another important measure of drugs effectiveness is its ability to prevent irreversible joint destruction as measured by radiographs. X-rays of hands and feet are obtained at predetermined intervals during a clinical trial. Using the

Sharp method [7] erosions and joint space narrowing are counted and scored in a blinded manner. Total Sharp scores are compared and used to determine radiographic progression.

Finally a patient's physical function can be measured at each visit using the disability index of the Health Assessment Questionnaire (HAQ) [8].

Several key studies have shown that adalimumab is effective in significantly improving the signs and symptoms of rheumatoid arthritis. Adalimumab has also been shown to slow the destructive potential of this disease as evidence by radiographic studies.

In an early study of patients with refractory rheumatoid arthritis several dose regiments of adalimumab as monotherapy were compared to placebo [9]. In this study, 284 patients 18 years old and over were randomized to receive either weekly injections of adalimumab 20 mg, 40 mg, 80 mg or placebo. To be eligible for enrollment patients needed to meet the revised 1987 American College of Rheumatology (ACR) criteria for the diagnosis of rheumatoid arthritis [10]. Patients were considered refractory to treatment if they failed at least one traditional DMARD and continued to have active synovitis as defined by more than 12 tender joints, more than 10 swollen joints and either an erythrocyte sedimentation rate (ESR) greater than 28 mm/h or C reactive protein (CRP) greater than 2.0 mg/l. Patients with recent surgery, hospitalization or infection were excluded.

All DMARDS were discontinued 4 weeks prior to starting either adalimumab or placebo. Non-steroidal anti-inflammatory drugs (NSAIDS) and corticosteroids (10 mg of prednisone or less) were allowed to be continued. The mean age of the subjects was 52.4 years and 79% were woman. The average patient had rheumatoid arthritis for 10.0 years and had taken 3.75 DMARDS in the past. All subjects were evaluated every 2 weeks over the 12-week study period. The primary endpoints were the number of subjects achieving an ACR 20 at week 12. Other evaluations included the number of subjects attaining an ACR 50 and ACR 70 as well as improvement in the disability index of the HAQ.

After 12 weeks of study 51% of patients taking 20 mg adalimumab, 57% of patients taking 40 mg of adalimumab and 54% of patients taking 80 mg of adalimumab reached an ACR 20 response. This response was statistically significantly higher than the 10% of patients taking placebo who attained an ACR 20 response. Improvement on adalimumab appeared quite rapid with 71% obtaining the ultimate ACR 20 response after 2 weeks of treatment.

ACR 50 responses were obtained in 24% Of patients taking the 20 mg dose of adalimumab, 27% of those taking the 40 mg dose and 19% of those taking the 80 mg dose. This response proved to be significantly higher than the 1% of patients taking placebo who obtained an ACR 50.

Finally an ACR 70 response was achieved in 11% of patients taking the 20 mg dose, 13% taking 40 mg and 8% taking 80 mg of adalimumab. These results also achieved significance as none of the patients taking placebo achieved an ACR 70.

All treatment groups also achieved a significant reduction in HAQ disability index scores when compared to placebo.

All doses of adalimumab were well tolerated. There were no significant differences in serious adverse reactions between treatment and placebo groups. Local injection site reactions (redness, itching, pain) did appear higher in the adalimumab groups.

In conclusion weekly doses of adalimumab as monotherapy in patients with rheumatoid arthritis who had failed previous DMARDS proved to be a safe and effective therapy. The 40 mg dose of adalimumab appeared to be equally effective as the 80 mg dose.

Based on the half-life of adalimumab a subsequent study looked at whether less frequent dosing of the medication would also prove to be effective [11]. Every other week dosing of adalimumab was compared to weekly dosing and placebo. Adalimumab was again given as monotherapy in patients with rheumatoid arthritis who had failed treatment with previous DMARDs.

In a 26 week study patients over 18 years old with active rheumatoid arthritis were randomized to receive either adalimumab 20 mg a week, 20 mg every other week, 40 mg a week, 40 mg every other week or placebo. 544 patients were enrolled in this study. The average age was 53 years and 77% were female. Patients had on average 11 years of disease and had taken 3.7 DMARDS. All DMARDS were discontinued 4 weeks prior to starting the study. Looking at ACR 20, 50 and 70 response rates as well as the HAQ disability index all patients receiving adalimumab had significant improvement when compared to placebo. The results suggested that the 40 mg doses provided better efficacy than the 20 mg doses. There was also the suggestion that 40 mg a week might offer some benefit over 40 mg every other week. All doses of adalimumab were well tolerated. Serious adverse event were similar to placebo. Again injection site reactions seemed to be higher in patients receiving adalimumab.

In conclusion this study showed that the current recommended dose of adalimumab (40 mg every other week) was safe and effective as monotherapy for rheumatoid arthritis. There may also be some patients who obtain some additional benefit by have the dose increased to 40 mg every week.

While the previous two studies have looked at adalimumab as monotherapy current practice in rheumatology has made it important to see whether adalimumab can be safely added to other DMARDS. Equally important is to determine whether such an addition can provide added benefit.

In recent years methotrexate has become one of the most established treatments for rheumatoid arthritis [12]. Nonetheless there are patients who continue to have active arthritis despite adequate doses of methotrexate. It has become common practice to add other DMARDS to methotrexate in the treatment of this disease [13].

In the ARMADA trial the addition of adalimumab to methotrexate used for treatment of rheumatoid arthritis was studied [14]. In this study 271 patients on established doses of methotrexate yet with active arthritis were randomized to receive adalimumab or placebo. Methotrexate in the dose at entry into the study was continued. On average patients were 55.5 years old and had disease duration of 12.3 years. The average weekly dose of methotrexate was 16.5 mg. Patients received either adalimumab 20 mg, 40 mg, 80 mg every other week or placebo and were studied for 24 weeks.

Analysis was made of ACR 20, 50 and 70 response rates as well as the HAQ disability index. At the conclusion of this study the patients who had adalimumab added to their methotrexate were significantly more improved than those taking methotrexate alone. There was the suggestion that those taking the 40 and 80 mg doses were most improved. The addition of adalimumab to methotrexate did not appear to significantly increase the risk of serious adverse events. Based on this study the addition of adalimumab to methotrexate appears to provide added benefit without added risk.

The preceding studies have looked at the effect of adalimumab on the signs and symptoms of rheumatoid arthritis. The ability of adalimumab to effect the radiographic progression and thus to modify the destructive potential of rheumatoid arthritis has also been studied [15]. In a 52 week study of patients with active rheumatoid arthritis despite treatment with methotrexate the ability of adalimumab to inhibit radiographic progression was analyzed. 619 patients with an average disease duration of 10.9 years taking methtrexate were randomized to have the addition of either adalimumab 40 mg every other week, 20 mg every week or placebo. X-rays of hands, wrists and feet were obtained at 24 and 52 weeks.

Patients receiving adalimumab had significantly fewer joint erosions ad significantly less joint space narrowing than those taking methotrexate alone. Despite long standing disease and previous DMARD therapy adalimumab was shown to be able to alter the natural history of this destructive disease.

In conclusion, a number of clinical trials have shown that adalimumab is a safe and effective treatment for rheumatoid arthritis. It can be used as monotherapy or in combination with other DMARDS in particular methotrexate. Patients taking adalimumab clinically improve and have a slowing of radiographic progression. The recommended dose is 40 mg by sc injection every other week. There may be some patients who obtain added benefit by increasing the dose to 40 mg every week.

References

1 Gabriel SE (2001) The epidemiology of rheumatoid arthritis. *Rheum Dis Clin North Am* 27: 269–281

2 Lard LR, Visser H, Speyer I, Vander Horst-Bruinsma IE, Zwinderman AH, Breedveld FC, Hazes JM (2001) Early *versus* delayed treatment in patients with recent-onset rheumatoid arthritis: comparison of two cohorts who received different treatment strategies. *Am J Med* 111: 446–451

3 O'Dell JR (2004) Therapeutic strategies for rheumatoid arthritis. *New Eng J Med* 350: 2591–2602

4 Olsen NJ, Stein CM (2004) New drugs for rheumatoid arthritis. *New Eng J Med* 350: 2167–2179

5 Saxne T, Palladino MA, Heinegard D, Talal N, Wollheim FA (1988) Detection of tumor necrosis

factor alpha but not tumor necrosis factor beta in rheumatoid arthritis synovial fluid and serum. *Arthritis Rheum* 31: 1041–1045
6 Choy EHS, Panayi GS (2001) Cytokine pathways and joint inflammation in rheumatoid arthritis. *New Eng J Med* 344: 907–916
7 Sharp JT, Young DY, Bluhm DY, Brook A, Brower AC, Corbett M, Decker JL, Genant HK, Gofton JP, Goodman N et al (1985) How many joints in the hands and wrists should be included in a score of radiologic progression in early rheumatoid arthritis clinical trials? *Arthritis Rheum* 28: 1326–1335
8 Fries JF, Spitz PW, Young DY (1982) The dimensions of health outcomes: the Health Assessment Questionnaire, disability and pain scales. *J Rheumatol* 9: 789–793
9 Van De Putte LBA, Rau R, Breedveld FC, Kalden JR, Malaise MG, Van Riel PLCM, Schattenkirchner M, Emery P, Burmester GR, Zeidler H et al (2003) Efficacy and safety of the fully human anti-tumour necrosis factor alpha monoclonal antibody adalimumab (D2E7) in DMARD refractory patients with rheumatoid arthritis: a 12-week phase II study. *Ann Rheum Dis* 1168–1177
10 Arnett FC, Edworthy SM, Bloch DA (1988) The American Rheumatism Association 1987 revised criteria for the classification of rheumatoid arthritis. *Arthritis Rheum* 31: 315–324
11 Van De Putte LBA, Atkins C, Malaise M, Sany J, Russel AS, Van Riel PLCM, Settas L, Bijlsma JW, Todesco S, Dougados M et al (2004) Efficacy and safety of adalimumab as monotherapy in patients with rheumatoid arthritis for whom previous disease modifying antirheumatic drug treatment has failed. *Ann Rheum Dis* 63: 508–516
12 Kremer JM (1997) Safety, efficacy, and mortality in a long-term cohort of patients with rheumatoid arthritis taking methotrexate: follow-up after a mean of 13.3 years. *Arthritis Rheum* 40: 984–985
13 Kremer JM (2001) Rational use of new and existing disease-modifying agents in rheumatoid arthritis. *Ann Intern Meed* 138: 695–706
14 Weinblatt ME, Keystone EC, Furst DE, Moreland LW, Weisman MH, Bibara CA, Teoh LA, Fischkoff SA, Chartash EK (2003) Adalimumab, a fully human anti-tumor necrosis factor alpha monoclonal antibody, for the treatment of rheumatoid arthritis in patients taking concomitant methotrexate The ARMADA trial. *Arthritis Rheum* 48: 35–45
15 Keystone EC, Kavanaugh AF, Sharp JT (2004) Radiographic, clinical, and functional outcomes of treatment with adalimumab (a human anti-tumor necrosis factor monoclonal antibody) in patients with active rheumatoid arthritis receiving concomitant methotrexate therapy. *Arthritis Rheum* 50: 1400–1411

TNF-alpha Inhibitors
Edited by Jeffrey M. Weinberg and Robin Buchholz

Adalimumab in dermatology

Jennifer Clay Cather and Melodie Young

Baylor University Medical Center, Dallas, Texas, USA

Introduction

Psoriasis and psoriatic arthritis are disease states of chronic inflammation mediated by T lymphocytes and the type 1 inflammatory cytokines they elaborate [1]. Psoriatic arthritis may be associated with disability and increased mortality [2]. While the true incidence of psoriatic arthritis is unknown, it has been estimated that between 10–30% of patients with psoriasis have psoriatic arthritis [2, 3]. Central to the pathogenesis of psoriasis is the proinflammatory cytokine tumor necrosis factor-alpha (TNF-α). Adalimumab (D2E7, Humira®; Abbott Laboratories, North Chicago, IL, USA) is a fully human monoclonal antibody directed against TNF-α. It is a self-administered subcutaneous injection approved in December 2002 by the Food and Drug Administration (FDA) in the United States (US) for the treatment of rheumatoid arthritis (RA) with or without concomitant methotrexate. It was approved for RA by the European Medicines Evaluation Agency in May 2003. Additionally, approval was obtained in Canada in September 2004 for the same indication. In the US, adalimumab has completed Phase III trials for psoriatic arthritis and filing with the FDA for this indication was submitted in December 2004. In July 2005 adalimumab was approved for the treatment of psoriatic arthritis in the US. We will review the findings in the pertinent psoriasis and psoriatic arthritis trials to date with emphasis on efficacy – safety is reviewed in the next chapter.

Clinical trials for psoriasis and psoriatic arthritis (Tab. 1)

Psoriatic arthritis

In an open label pilot study, patients with psoriatic arthritis treated with 40 mg subcutaneous every other week showed significant improvement [4]. Soon thereafter, in a large double-blind randomized controlled trial (ADEPT) patients (n = 313) were treated with placebo (n = 162) or 40 mg of adalimumab subcutaneously every other week (n = 151) (Fig. 1). In both treatment groups, 50% of patients continued their stable doses of methotrexate (50% of

Table 1 Clinical trials for psoriasis and psoriatic arthritis

	Psoriatic arthritis	
Trial	Phase	Design
Open label	Pilot	Open label pilot study (n = 15)
M02-518 (ADEPT)	III	24-week double blind placebo control study (n = 313)
M02-537	III	120-week open label extension for patients completing M02-518
	Psoriasis	
Trial	Phase	Design
M02-528	II	12 week double blind placebo control with 2 active dosing arms (n = 147)
M02-529	II	48-week extension study for patients completing M02-528. (n = 137)
M02-538	II	76-week randomized trial (n = 148)

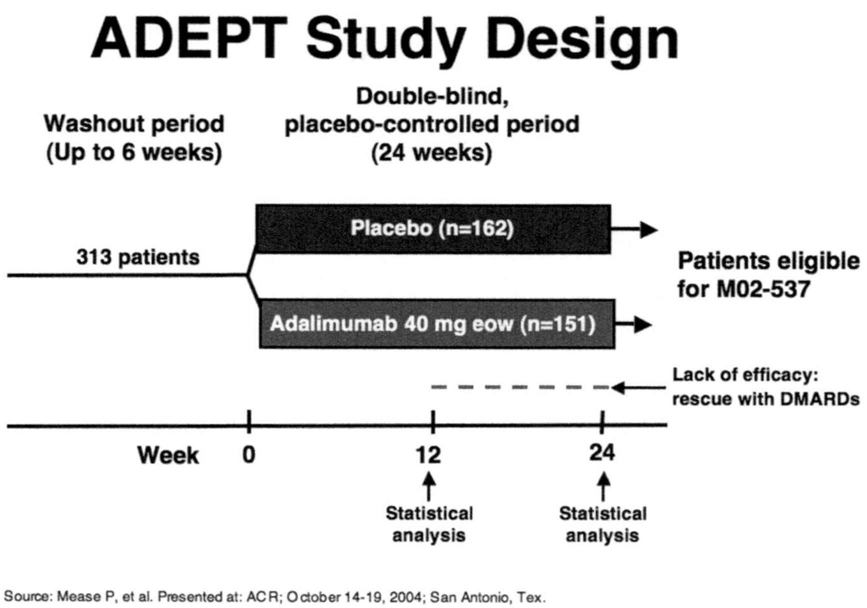

Figure 1. Adalimumab in Psoriatic Arthritis (ADEPT trial).

the placebo group and 51% of the adalimumab group). The ACR 20/50/70 responses at 6 months were 57%/39%/23% for adalimumab and 15%/6%/1% in the placebo group ($p < 0.001$) [5]. Quality of life improved and disability decreased in patients who received adalimumab. Recently, at EULAR 2005, the radiographic data from the ADEPT trial was presented by Mease et al. in poster form. At 24 weeks (placebo control part of study) there was no radiographic progression in the adalimumab treated patients and this response was maintained at 48 weeks (open label extension). Additionally, Kavanaugh et al. presented in poster form at EULAR 2005 the finding that responses were the same with or without concomitant methotrexate.

Psoriasis

In all the psoriasis trials discussed below, chronic plaque psoriasis was required for entry and no concomitant systemic medications were allowed for the treatment of psoriasis. At entry, patients in these studies were naïve to TNF inhibitor therapy. The initial phase II study (M02-528) was a randomized double-blind placebo controlled trial in which two different dosing arms were compared to placebo (Fig. 2). Prior to baseline, the following washout periods were required: 2 weeks for topicals and phototherapy, 4 weeks for nonbiologic systemic therapies, and 12 weeks for biologics. In one treatment arm

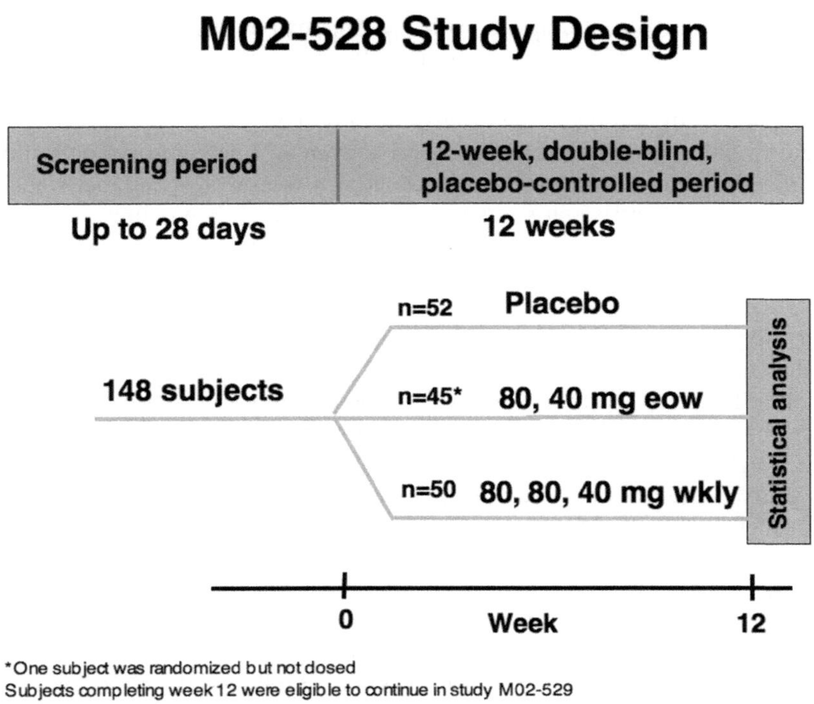

Figure 2. Adalimumab in Psoriasis (M02–528).

(n = 45) patients received 80 mg adalimumab at week 0 and then received 40 mg every other week starting at week 1. In the other treatment arm (n = 50), patients received 80 mg adalimumab at week 0 and 1 and then 40 mg every week starting at week 2. There were 52 patients in the placebo group. The results were recently presented in poster form at the American Academy of Dermatology Meeting in February 2004. Clinical responses were rapid (clinically statistically different from placebo at week 1) and sustained over the dosing period. At week 12 the PASI 75 rates for placebo, every other week, and weekly dosing were 4%, 53%, and 80%, respectively [6, 7]. An extension study (M02-529) was available for the 132 patients who completed M02-528 in which the patients previously on placebo (n = 47) received 80 mg adalimumab at week 12 and then 40 mg every other week (eow) starting at week 13 up to week 48. Patients who received active drug in the previous study were continued for an additional 48 weeks in their previously randomized dosing groups – every other week (n = 45) or weekly dosing (n = 50) for an additional 48 weeks. The long-term (529) data was recently presented by Dr Richard Langley in a poster at the 24th Anniversary Fall Clinical Dermatology Conference 2005. Once again, the clinical response in the placebo group was rapid and sustained with 55% of patients obtaining a PASI 75 after 12 weeks of 40 mg eow dosing. Longer time on therapy did not improve the efficacy of the group receiving weekly dosing; however, efficacy was sustained and after a total of 60 weeks of therapy, 64% of patients had a PASI 75. On the other hand, the every other week dosing group efficacy peaked after 24 total weeks of dosing and was sustained with 58% of patients obtaining a PASI 75 at week 60. 31 patients discontinued the extension study. The primary reasons for premature discontinuation were: 9 for adverse events, 9 per protocol definition (i.e., did not achieve a PASI 50 response after 8 weeks of open label weekly therapy), 6 for unsatisfactory therapeutic effect, and 2 withdrew consent. Adverse events leading to discontinuation are listed in Table 2.

Durability of response was evaluated by a Phase II randomized trial (M02-538) in which all 148 patients received open label adalimumab (80 mg week 0 and 1 followed by 40 mg every week starting at week 2) for the first 12 weeks and then the PASI 50 responders entered in a randomized, double-blind, placebo-controlled period. During the double-blind placebo control period, patients received placebo (n = 68) or 40 mg of adalimumab every other week (n = 68) for 12 weeks. Thereafter, patients were seen 4 weeks after their last dose and then every 3 months until relapse or week 76. After the initial 12 weeks of open label dosing, 91.9% of patients (n = 136) achieved at least a PASI50, 76.4% (n = 113) achieved a PASI75 and 47.3% (n = 70) reached a PASI90. At week 12, patients were randomized to placebo or every other week dosing. There was a low rate of relapse (defined as <PASI50) between weeks 12–24 for both the placebo and every other week dosing groups, 31% (n = 21) and 16% (n = 11) respectively. There were no cases of rebound in either treatment group (rebound was defined as an increase in PASI by 125% or development of generalized or pustular psoriasis). Discontinuations were primarily due to

Table 2 Serious adverse events leading to discontinuation in adalimumab trials for PsA and Ps

Study	Event
M02-518 (ADEPT)	Judged as possibly related to study drug by investigator: Viral meningitis (West Nile virus)
M02-528 Weeks 0-12	All judged as unrelated to study drug by investigators: Metastatic squamous cell carcinoma (40 mg eow) Cerebrovascular accident (40 mg qw) 70 days after last dose Migraine (40 mg qw) Bronchitis (40 mg qw) Breast carcinoma (40 mg qw) 5 weeks after initiation of drug
M02-529 Weeks 12-60	Judged as possibly related or unrelated: Malignant melanoma (40 mg eow) appeared under a resolving psoriasis plaque Malignant melanoma (40 mg wk) within a tattoo Gastric adenocarcinoma (40 mg qw) Palpitations (40 mg qw) Hematocrit abnormal (40 mg eow) Coccidioidomycosis (40 mg eow) Conversion of TB skin test – no active TB (40 mg wk) Psoriatic arthropathy (40 mg eow) ALT/AST elevated (40 mg wk)
M02-538	Both judged as unrelated to study drug by investigators: Diverticulitis (40 mg wk/40 mg eow) Post-op wound infection (40 mg wk/40 mg eow)

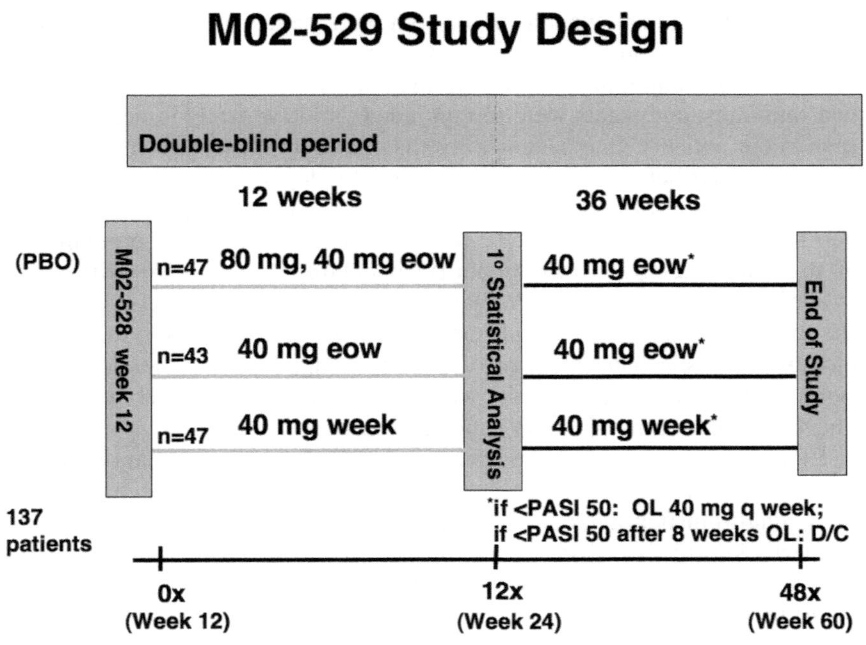

Figure 3. Adalimumab Psoriasis Extension Study (M02–529).

relapse (n = 32); however, two serious adverse events occurred which lead to treatment discontinuation (see Tab. 2). The Phase III trial is ongoing.

Clinical experience

The first published experience using adalimumab for the treatment of psoriasis and psoriatic arthritis was reported by Chew et al. in 2004 [8]. These authors reported two patients with refractory psoriasis who both improved after initiation of adalimumab (40 mg sq every other week). Of note, one patient had erythrodermic psoriasis that had become unresponsive to infliximab (discontinuation resulted from a loss of clinical efficacy and a delayed infusion reaction). It has been noted in the Crohn's population that adalimumab may be effective and well tolerated in patients who have lost their response or are intolerant of infliximab [9, 10]. Additionally, in patients with Crohn's who develop allergic reactions to infliximab, and even a small number of patients who developed infliximab-induced lupus, tolerated adalimumab and benefited from therapy [11]. An increasing number of published reports described successful treatment of plaque psoriasis with adalimumab [12].

At Texas Dermatology Associates we have treated over 60 psoriasis patients with and without psoriatic arthritis with adalimumab in a variety of dosing regimens (monotherapy weekly, monotherapy every other week, and combination therapy with traditional immunosuppressants). Some of our patients were previously on infliximab, etanercept, or both with inadequate clinical responses. Adequate disease control with respect to skin and joints symptoms was accomplished with adalimumab in most. In the majority of patients, their concomitant immunosuppressants were discontinued. No new safety issues have been seen in our patients. One patient who was on concomitant cyclosporine developed an ocular herpes infection. The ophthalmologist elected to continue the cyclosporine and discontinue the adalimumab. One other patient developed dermatomal herpes simplex. One patient who was previously on etanercept 50 mg twice weekly for over 6 months had obtained good control with respect to her joints; however, only minimal cutaneous clearing was seen. As a result, she discontinued etanercept and started weekly adalimumab. On follow-up, 2 months later, she had evidence of skin clearing; however, her joints were symptomatically and functionally worse. As a result, adalimumab was discontinued after 4 months of therapy and etanercept was restarted.

Psoriatic onycho-pachydermo periostitis (POPP) is a rare variant of psoriatic arthritis (world-wide cases reported = 15) which is clinically characterized by digital drumstick-like deformity resulting from psoriatic onychodystrophy, connective tissue thickening above the distal phalanx, and periosteal reaction [13]. This disease is associated with a great deal of pain and functional impairment. In general, improvement with traditional DMARDs has been minimal; however, in one case there was a dramatic improvement 10 days after one subcutaneous 40 mg adalimumab injection [13]. Clinical efficacy was maintained on every other week dosing for over 4 months. After 4 months of therapy, nails and digits appeared normal as well as repeat magnetic resonance imaging (MRI) studies.

Other uses

Of anecdotal interest, one patient with Crohn's who developed morphea was treated with adalimumab 40 mg every other week. Previously, she had an infusion reaction on infliximab. After introduction of adalimumab, the patient reported subjective improvement of her Crohn's with no associated improvement in her morphea after 4 months of therapy (personal observation of Jennifer Cather MD and Melissa Costner MD). She remains on adalimumab for Crohn's.

Conclusion

Adalimumab will be a welcomed addition to our psoriasis armamentarium. The data with respect to efficacy, safety, and quality of life in both psoriatic arthritis and psoriasis are promising.

Acknowledgements
Thank you to Jennifer Henkes for supplying trial schematics and for forwarding articles. Thank you to Rebecca Hoffman for clarifying adverse events reported in clinical trials. Thanks to Alan Menter and William Abramovits who we formally worked with at Texas Dermatology Associates for the good times we had in the psoriasis clinic.

References

1 Krueger JG (2002) The immunologic basis for the treatment of psoriasis with new biologic agents. *J Am Acad Dermatol* 46: 1–23
2 Gladman DD (2004) Psoriatic arthritis. *Dermatol Ther* 17(5): 350–363
3 Mease PJ (2005) Psoriatic arthritis therapy advances. *Curr Opin Rheumatol* 17(4): 426–432
4 Ritchlin C, Anandarajaha A, Tolterman S, Shao T, Kemshati S, Badger W, Durham R (2004) Preliminary data from a study of adalimumab in the treatment of psoriatic arthritis. *Ann Rheum Dis* 63 (suppl 1): 403
5 Mease PJ, Gladman DD, Ritchlin CT, Ruderman EM, Steinfeld SD, Choy EH, Sharp JT, Ory PA, Perdok RJ, Weinberg MA (2004) Adalimumab effectiveness in psoriatic arthritis trial study group: 24-week results of a phase III study. *Arthritis Rheum* 50: 4097
6 Chen DM, Gordon KB, Leonardi C, Menter AM (2004) Adalimumab efficacy and safety in patients with moderate to severe chronic plaque psoriasis: prelimimary findings from a 12-week dose ranging trial. *J Am Acad Dermatol* 50: S1
7 Patel T, Gordon K (2004) Adalimumab: efficacy and safety in psoriasis and rheumatoid arthritis. *Dermatologic Therapy* 17: 427–431
8 Chew AL, Bennett A, Smith CH, Barker J, Kirkham B (2004) Successful treatment of psoriasis and psoriatic arthritis with adalimumab. *Br J Dermatol* 151(2): 492–496
9 Sandborn WJ, Hanauer S, Loftus EV Jr, Tremaine WJ, Kane S, Cohen R, Hanson K, Johnson T, Schmitt D, Jeche R (2004) An open-label study of the human anti-TNF monoclonal antibody adalimumab in subjects with prior loss of response or intolerance to infliximab for Crohn's disease.

Am J Gastroenterol 99: 1984–1989
10 Papadakis KA, Shaye OA, Vasiliauskas EA, Ippoliti A, Dubinsky MC, Birt J, Paavola J, Lee SK, Price J, Targan SR, Abreu MT (2005) Safety and efficacy of adalimumab (D2E7) in Crohn's disease patients with an attenuated response to infliximab. *Am J Gastroenterol* 100: 75–79
11 Youdim A, Vasiliauskas EA, Targan SR, Papadakis KA, Ippoliti A, Dubinsky MC, Lechago J, Paavola J, Loane J, Lee SK et al (2004) A pilot study of adalimumab in infliximab-allergic patients. *Inflammatory Bowel Disorder* 10: 333–338
12 Sladden MJ, Mortimer NJ, Hutchinson PE (2005) Extensive plaque psoriasis successfully treated with adalimumab (Humira). *Br J Dermatol* 152(5): 1091–1092
13 Bongartz T, Harle P, Friedrich S, Karrer S, Vogt T, Seitz A, Muller-Ladner U (2005) Successful treatment of psoriatic onycho-pachydermo periostitis (POPP) with adalimumab. *Arthritis Rheum* 52(1): 280–282

TNF-alpha Inhibitors
Edited by Jeffrey M. Weinberg and Robin Buchholz

A review of the safety of the tumor necrosis inhibitors infliximab, etanercept, and adalimumab

Jeffrey M. Weinberg

Department of Dermatology, St. Luke's-Roosevelt Hospital Center and Beth Israel Medical Center, New York, USA

Summary

The TNF-inhibitors infliximab, etanercept, and adalimumab share a number of common safety issues and concerns. There is an increased risk of reactivation of granulomatous diseases, especially tuberculosis, with all three agents and appropriate steps should be taken for detection and treatment of latent infections. In terms of malignancy, an association between non-Hodgkin's lymphoma and treatment with TNF-antagonists has been reported, although patients with active, long-standing rheumatoid arthritis (RA) and psoriasis have been reported to have an increased incidence this condition. The biological plausability of lymphomas associated with immunomodulatory agents raises concern and vigilance is recommended until the relationship is fully characterized. Large phase II and III trials have shown a negative effect of TNF-inhibitors in advanced heart failure and these agents should be avoided in this population. Rare case reports of drug-induced lupus, seizure disorder, pancytopenia, and demyelinating diseases have been noted after use of these agents and continued vigilance is warranted in patients on TNF-antagonists for the development of these diseases. Currently there is no evidence implicating TNF-inhibitors with embryotoxicity, teratogenicity or increased pregnancy loss.

Infections

General bacterial infections

In the clinical trials, the use of all three TNF-antagonists was associated with bacterial infections requiring treatment. Most of the infections were minor, treated with either outpatient antibiotic therapy and/or temporary withdrawal of the drug. The most commonly reported infections were those of the respiratory tract (including sinusitis, pharyngitis, and bronchitis) and the urinary tract.

In the infliximab clinical studies, treated infections were reported in 36% of patients on infliximab compared with 26% in the placebo-treated group [1]. The risk of serious infections (requiring hospitalizations or parenteral antibiotics) in the infliximab studies for both Crohn's disease and RA was 6.2% compared with 6.8% in the placebo group (Crohn's disease 5.2% in the infliximab group *versus* 1.8% in the placebo group, RA 8.1% in the infliximab *versus* 9.0% in the placebo group) [2]. In trials comparing etanercept and placebo, 35% of patients in the treatment group developed infections compared with 32% in the placebo group [3]. In trials comparing etanercept plus methotrexate to methotrexate alone, 64% in the etanercept group developed an infection compared with 72% in the methotrexate group. Serious infections occurred in 1% of the patients in both the etanercept and placebo groups [3]. In adalimumab studies, 52.7% adalimumab patients developed infections compared with 46.7% in the placebo group. The incidence of serious infections was 1.7% in the adalimumab group *versus* 1.4% in the placebo group [4]. The risk of serious infections in RA patients in the pre-TNF-antagonist era was 0.03–0.09 cases/patient-year [5, 6]. The incidence of serious infections in the clinical trials with TNF-antagonists is as follows: etanercept 0.04/patient-year [3], adalimumab 0.04/patient-year [4], and infliximab 0.06/patient-year [7].

In summary, TNF-antagonists are associated with an increased risk of serious infections compared with the general population but the rate is similar to RA patients treated with other disease-modifying agents in the pre-TNF era. When serious infections occur, TNF-antagonists should not be started or should be discontinued [7]. Treatment with these agents can be resumed after the infections have been treated adequately [8].

Tuberculosis

Infection is an issue of major concern, and there have been multiple reports of reactivation of latent tuberculosis with infliximab (TB) [9–11]. The available *in vitro* and epidemiological evidence for the TNF inhibitors infliximab and etanercept shows that the risk of development of active tuberculosis is higher with infliximab [12]. In controlled trials, however, an increased risk of serious infection in infliximab-treated patients has not been observed [9].

Even though there were only two cases of tuberculosis reported in clinical trials of infliximab [1] there have been 295 cases of infliximab-associated tuberculosis reported as of August 2002 [7, 13]. This gives an estimated rate of 37 cases per 100,000 (86 cases/233,547 exposed) and 150 cases per 100,000 in Europe (156 cases/103,335 exposed) [7]. As of March 2002, 36 tuberculosis cases/~150,000 treated have been reported with etanercept giving a rate of approximately 24 cases per 100,000 patients treated [7]. In comparison, the background rate of tuberculosis in RA patients in the US is estimated to be 6.2 cases per 100,000 person [13] and 20 cases per 100,000 person [14] in Europe.

In a detailed evaluation of 70 cases of tuberculosis treated with infliximab [10] it was found that 56 of these had extrapulmonary tuberculosis, and 79% of the cases received one or more concurrent medications (corticosteroids alone or in combination with methotrexate). The median interval from start of infliximab to onset of tuberculosis was 12 weeks (range 1–52 weeks). Interestingly, 91% of the cases were from countries with a low incidence of tuberculosis. Suggestion of an association between treatment with infliximab and development of tuberculosis is strengthened by the close temporal association to infliximab administration, the higher estimated rate of tuberculosis compared with the background rates in RA patients, and the laboratory evidence linking susceptibility to tuberculosis with decreases in TNF activity [10].

Mohan et al. [15] reviewed 25 cases of TB due to etanercept, which were reported to the US Food and Drug Administration (FDA) between November 1998 and March 2002. 15 patients received other immunosuppressive medications. The median interval between the receipt of the first dose of etanercept and the diagnosis of TB was 11.5 months. 13 patients had extrapulmonary TB at the time of diagnosis. Diagnosis was made on the basis of culture results for 12 patients, biopsy findings for 9, and sputum staining for 4. There were 2 deaths, 1 of which was directly attributed to TB. The estimated number of TB cases reported to the FDA for each person-year of treatment with etanercept (i.e., the 'reporting rate') among patients with rheumatoid arthritis (RA) was ~10 cases/100,000 patient-years of exposure. The authors concluded that clinicians considering etanercept for patients with RA should be alert to the possibility of the occurrence of TB, sometimes with an unusual extrapulmonary presentation. It is unclear whether etanercept therapy increases the risk of TB beyond the elevated TB rates already documented for patients with RA [15].

There were 13 cases of tuberculosis seen with adalimumab during 4,870 patient-years of clinical trials; most of these cases occurred within the first 8 months of initiation of therapy [4]. Eight of these cases occurred in the Phase I and II development program where supratherapeutic doses were used. During the Phase III study, where the 40 mg every other week dose (currently approved FDA dose for the treatment of RA) was used and tuberculosis prophylaxis was instituted, five more cases occurred [7].

Although postmarketing cases of tuberculosis have been reported for both etanercept and infliximab, the data suggest, but do not prove, that the risk of tuberculosis is different for the two agents. In voluntary reporting systems, the reporting rate among infliximab users is several-fold higher than the incidence in the general US population. In addition, more cases of tuberculosis have been seen among patients not otherwise considered at risk of tuberculosis. Tuberculosis has also been seen in the clinical trials of infliximab and adalimumab. These findings led to a black box warning by the FDA in the infliximab and adalimumab inserts [1, 4]. Etanercept has a bold warning, but no black box warning regarding tuberculosis [3]. For etanercept, postmarketing cases of tuberculosis have been uncommon, with a reporting rate similar to or a little higher than the US incidence. Most patients who developed tuberculosis were considered to be at high risk for other reasons. Also, no cases of tuberculosis have been seen through October 2002 in etanercept trial of patients with RA either in the US or Europe (tota1 3,280 patients) In North America, the purified protein derivative (PPD) is usually used to screen for tuberculosis, but some questions about this practice, rather than chest films, have recently been raised.

Reactivation of tuberculosis can occur with TNF antagonists. Patients should be evaluated with a PPD test and/or a chest x-ray, if needed [16]. Patients with evidence of latent tuberculosis should be treated before TNF blocking agents are used [16]. PPD skin test criteria for patient receiving TNF antagonists have recently been published [12]. Some authorities suggest that TNF antagonists may be started as soon as antituberculosis treatment is started, although this approach needs further evaluation.

Hamilton [17] recently reviewed the infectious complications of biologic therapy. His review described the most important pathogen-specific infections and their relative frequency. Tuberculosis has continued to be the most common pathogen reported in association with infliximab, and less so with etanercept and adalimumab. Determining treated population case rates depends on having an accurate denominator and reflects the local population's latent infection rate. The same is true for histoplasmosis. Other pathogens requiring intact cellular immunity for control of latent infection have also been reported. Specific recommendations for preventive therapy are being made, but prospective clinical trials are needed to assess the risk–benefit of any particular approach. He concluded that microorganisms responsible for the infectious complications associated with anticytokine therapy are generally intracellular pathogens or pathogens that commonly exist in a chronic, latent state and are normally held in check by cell-mediated immunity. Diagnosis requires a high index of suspicion and prompt acquisition of appropriate tissue for microscopic examination and microbiologic culture [17].

Fungal and viral infections

Patients treated with TNF-α antagonists, especially infliximab, may have an increased risk of reactivation of granulomatous fungal infections [18]. Therefore, patients living in high-risk areas should be monitored closely. Unlike tuberculosis, guidelines have not been developed to screen or treat latent fungal infection before initiating the anti-TNF-α therapy. Many opportunistic infections have been reported but their incidence is extremely low. When considering infections where host defenses are particularly macrophage dependent, physicians should exercise careful vigilance, especially in areas of high disease prevalence, while using anti-TNF-α agent [18].

There is a paucity of data suggesting that TNF-α antagonists predispose to an increased incidence of viral infections, although their mechanism of action should make one keep this possibility in mind when treating patients with the TNF-α antagonists [18]. Preliminary evidence suggests a beneficial role of the TNF-α antagonists in hepatitis C. TNF-α antagonists should be used very carefully in patients with HIV (for fear of activation of infections) and probably avoided in the hepatitis B carrier state due to the risk of reactivation of their hepatitis B.

Lymphoma

One of the major concerns with the use of TNF inhibitors is the potential risk for development of lymphomas. Brown et al. [19] investigated the occurrence of lymphoproliferative disorders in patients treated with these agents. They reviewed relevant data in the MedWatch postmarket adverse event surveillance system run by the US FDA and identified 26 cases of lymphoproliferative disorders following treatment with etanercept (18 cases) or infliximab (8 cases). The majority of cases (81%) were non-Hodgkin's lymphomas. The interval between initiation of therapy with etanercept or infliximab and the development of lymphoma was very short (median 8 weeks). The authors concluded that, although data from a case series such theirs cannot establish a clear causal relationship between exposure to these medications and the risk of lymphoproliferative disease, the known predisposition of patients with diseases such as RA and CD to lymphoma, the known excess of lymphoma in other immunosuppressed populations, and the known immunosuppressive effects of the anti-TNF drugs, provide a biologic basis for concern and justification for the initiation of additional epidemiologic studies to formally evaluate this possible association [19].

The risk of lymphoma is increased in patients with rheumatoid arthritis (RA), and spontaneous reporting suggests that methotrexate (MTX) and anti-tumor necrosis factor (anti-TNF) therapy might be associated independently with an increased risk of lymphoma [20]. Wolfe and Michaud [20] conducted a study to determine the rate of and standardized incidence ratio (SIR) for lymphoma in patients with RA and in RA patient subsets by treatment group. Additionally, they sought to determine predictors of lymphoma in RA. They prospectively studied 18,572 patients with RA who were enrolled in the National Data Bank for Rheumatic Diseases (NDB). Patients were surveyed biannually, and potential lymphoma cases received detailed follow up. The SEER (Survey, Epidemiology, and End Results) cancer data resource was used to derive the expected number of cases of lymphoma in a cohort that was comparable in age and sex with the RA cohort [20].

The overall SIR for lymphoma was 1.9 (95% confidence interval [95% CI] 1.3–2.7). The SIR for biologic use was 2.9 (95% CI 1.7–4.9) and for the use of infliximab (with or without etanercept) was 2.6 (95% CI 1.4–4.5). For etanercept, with or without infliximab, the SIR was 3.8 (95% CI 1.9–7.5). The SIR for MTX was 1.7 (95% CI 0.9–3.2), and was 1.0 (95% CI 0.4–2.5) for those not receiving MTX or biologics. Lymphoma was associated with increasing age, male sex, and education. The authors concluded that lymphomas are increased in RA. Although the SIR is greatest for anti-TNF therapies, differences between therapies are slight, and confidence intervals for treatment groups overlap. The increased lymphoma rates observed with anti-TNF therapy may reflect channeling bias, whereby patients with the highest risk of lymphoma preferentially receive anti-TNF therapy. Current data are insufficient to establish a causal relationship between RA treatments and the development of lymphoma [20].

Adams et al. [21] described two cases of cutaneous and systemic T cell lymphoma that progressed rapidly in the setting of TNF-α blockade, one with etanercept and one with infliximab. Both cases were characterized by rapid onset, a fulminant clinical course with extensive cutaneous and systemic involvement, and death within months of diagnosis.

A warning was recently added to infliximab's package insert [22]. Data from studies showed a six-fold lymphoma increase among rheumatoid arthritis and Crohn's disease patients taking the drug. The studies showed a three-fold increase among arthritis patients alone. The studies suggest that the combined population of rheumatoid arthritis and Crohn's disease patients taking infliximab will have 12 cases of lymphoma for every 10,000 patients taking the drug for 1 year. Among arthritis patients alone, there would be seven lymphoma cases for every 10,000 patients taking infliximab for 1 year [22].

The incidence of lymphomas seen in patients receiving adalimumab is similar to that of the general RA population. Among 2,468 rheumatoid arthritis patients treated in clinical trials with the drug for a median of 24 months, 10 patients with lymphoma were seen. The Standardized Incidence Ratio (SIR) (ratio of observed rate to age-adjusted expected frequency in the general population) for lymphomas was 5.4 (95% CI, 2.6, 10.0) [23].

Demyelinating disease

There have been infrequent reports of central nervous system (CNS) demyelinating disorders during treatment with anti-TNF agents. Several of these cases have been temporally related to anti-TNF therapy and have resolved when treatment was withdrawn [24]. Mohan et al. [24] reviewed the occurrence of neurologic events suggestive of demyelination during anti-tumor necrosis factor alpha (anti-TNF) therapy for inflammatory arthritides. The Adverse Events Reporting System of the Food and Drug Administration (FDA) was queried following a report of a patient with refractory rheumatoid arthritis who developed confusion and difficulty with walking after receiving etanercept for 4 months. 19 patients with similar neurologic events were identified from the FDA database, 17 following etanercept administration and 2 following infliximab administration for inflammatory arthritis. All neurologic events were temporally related to anti-TNF therapy, with partial or complete resolution on discontinuation. One patient exhibited a positive rechallenge phenomenon. The authors concluded that further surveillance and studies are required to better define risk factors for and frequency of adverse events and their relationship to anti-TNF therapies. Until more long-term safety data are available, consideration should be given to avoiding anti-TNF therapy in patients with pre-existing multiple sclerosis and to discontinuing anti-TNF therapy immediately when new neurologic signs and symptoms occur, pending an appropriate evaluation [24].

Given this data, etanercept, infliximab, or adalimumab should be avoided in patients with a personal history of any CNS demyelinating disorder and used with caution in patients with a family history of these disorders.

Heart failure

There have been rare reports of heart failure in patients receiving anti-TNF therapy, but the relationship to therapy is unclear because the background rate of heart failure may be elevated in the patient populations receiving these drugs [25]. Kwon et al. [25], utilizing the US FDA's MedWatch program, documented 47 patients, who developed new or worsening heart failure during TNF antagonist therapy. After TNF antagonist therapy, 38 patients (26 etanercept, 12 infliximab) developed new-onset heart failure and 9 patients (3 etanercept, 6 infliximab) experienced heart failure exacerbation. Of the 38 patients with new-onset heart failure, 19 (50%) (12 etanercept, 7 infliximab) had no identifiable risk factors. The authors concluded that, in a fraction of patients, TNF antagonists might induce new-onset heart failure or exacerbate existing disease. However, they noted that these spontaneous reports alone are not sufficient to make causal inferences [25].

Drug-induced lupus

Induction of antinuclear (ANA) and anti-DNA antibodies is observed in some patients treated with infliximab and etanercept [26]. Recently, the induction of true lupus erythematosus by TNF-inhibitors has been observed. Few cases without major organ involvement were reported to be associated with infliximab treatment that resolved after anti-TNF discontinuation, [26–29] and only four cases have been described with the use of etanercept [30].

In the ATTRACT trial, 62% of patients developed a positive antinuclear antibody (ANA) compared with 27% of placebo-treated patients. Anti-double-stranded DNA (dsDNA) developed in 15% of infliximab-treated patients compared with none in the placebo arm. Most of the anti-dsDNA associated with infliximab are of IgM isotype. In the clinical studies, 6 patients developed systemic lupus erythematosus-like syndrome, which improved on stopping the biological therapy [1]. Children (n = 24) with a variety of rheumatological diseases were treated with infliximab. A total of 16.7% (4/24) of the patients developed anti-dsDNA antibodies during treatment with infliximab; however, none of them developed clinical signs and symptoms of systemic lupus erythematosus [31]. Longitudinal assessments of ANA and antibodies against dsDNA were done during the regulatory approval process for etanercept. During 6-month clinical trials, 11% of 323 patients treated with etanercept became positive for ANA, and 15% and 3% developed antibodies against dsDNA by radioimmunoassay and *Crithidia luciliae* assay, respectively, compared with 5% for ANA and 4% and none in the placebo group, respectively; no patients, however, developed clinical autoimmune disease [3].

22 case reports of lupus-like syndromes have recently been reported with etanercept in the form of case reports, series and FDAs AERS [30, 32].

Adalimumab has a 12% rate of positive ANA compared with placebo (7%). No data on dsDNA have been reported. One patient developed systemic lupus erythematosus-like syndrome and improved on discontinuation of the drug [4]. Most cases of drug-induced lupus with TNF-antagonists had skin and pleuropericardial involvement along with positive anti-dsDNA, anti-Smith and/or anti-histone antibodies as their manifestation [30, 32]. No patient thus far has developed neurological or renal disease.

In summary, patients treated with TNF-antagonists have an increased incidence of developing a positive ANA and dsDNA. Although antibodies develop to all TNF-antagonists, they may develop more frequently to infliximab, a chimeric antibody. The presence of these antibodies does not presage systemic lupus erythematosus-like disease (which is rare and reversible) and does not preclude their use.

Injection site/infusion reactions

Injection site reactions (ISRs) have been seen with both etanercept and adalimumab in their clinical trials. Etanercept was associated with ISRs in 37% of patients *versus* 7% in the placebo arm [33]. 7% of patients experienced redness at previous injection sites when subsequent injections were given [3]. None of the patients discontinued the drug due to ISRs. The ISRs usually occur in the first month of treatment and decrease with time. The reactions are believed to be T-lymphocyte-mediated, delayed-type hypersensitivity reactions which decrease in intensity over time possibly due to induced tolerance [34]. Adalimumab had 20.9% ISRs *versus* 14% in the placebo arm in the clinical trials [35]. ISRs cause 0.3% of patients to discontinue the drug, which was the same as in the placebo group.

Infliximab was associated with a 22% infusion reaction rate *versus* 9% in the placebo arm in their clinical studies. An infusion reaction was defined as any adverse event occurring during an infusion or within 2 h after infusion. Among 935 patients treated in clinical trials, 3% patients had nonspecific fever and chills, <1% of infusions were serious, which included anaphylaxis and hypotension [1]. Only 2.5% discontinued treatment due to these reactions in clinical trials [2].

In summary, ISRs are common with both etanercept and adalimumab and usually occur in the first month of treatment and decrease with time. Infliximab is associated with mild infusion reactions requiring either a decrease in the rate of infusion or pretreatment with a histamine H1 receptor antagonist, with or without low-dose parenteral glucocorticoids. Patients with anaphylactic reactions to infliximab should not receive another dose of infliximab.

Immunogenicity

Treatment with TNF antagonists can be associated with the formation of antibodies against the individual agents. An average of 10% of RA patients develops human anti-chimeric antibodies (HACA) to infliximab [1]. The presence of the antibody is associated with a higher rate of infusion reactions (defined as reaction occurring within 2 h of infusion). Among 25 patients with HACA and 125 controls without HACA, infusion reactions occurred in 11% of HACA-positive patients and 3% HACA-negative patients while American College of Rheumatology (ACR) 20% response was equal for the two groups (from the ATTRACT study) [6]. In a recent prospective study, 125 patients with Crohn's disease receiving infliximab infusion 5 mg/kg for the first time were evaluated for antibodies to infliximab and their relationship to infusion reactions and clinical efficacy [36]. There were technical issues relating to the antibody assay as well clinical problems relating to the definition of clinically important antibody concentrations, making associations between the presence and concentration of antibody and efficacy or toxicity very tenuous. Also, cut points for significant titers of antibodies were chosen ex *post facto* and arbitrarily. Beyond that, however, a high percentage of patients (approximately 47%) developed HACA in the Crohn's disease population after a single infusion. Concomitant use of immunosuppressives reduced the apparent immunogenic response.

In adalimumab clinical trials, 5% of RA patients developed antibodies to adalimumab. Patients using concomitant methotrexate had a lower rate of antibody formation than patients using the drug as monotherapy (1% *versus* 12%). The ACR 20% response was numerically but not statistically lower among antibody-positive patients than antibody-negative patients (30% *versus* 50%, $p = 0.1$) [7].

In etanercept clinical trials, <5% of patients developed antibodies, all of which were non-neutralizing [3]. Results were similar with psoriatic arthritis, ankylosing spondylitis and juvenile RA [3].

Infliximab, a chimeric antibody, clearly results in a higher incidence of HACA. The implication of this difference on efficacy is unclear, although these antibodies are associated with increased adverse events in some cases. Concomitant use of methotrexate reduces immunogenic response to both infliximab and adalimumab [1, 7].

Hematological: Aplastic anaemia, pancytopenia

Four cases of aplastic anaemia have been reported with the use of etanercept as of September 2001 [37]. The historical background incidence is 5.7–8.2 patients/100,000 patient-years with an increased incidence of aplastic anaemia in RA (odds ratio = 7.6, 95% CI 2.6, 23). 15 and 12 cases of pancytopenia have been reported with infliximab and etanercept, respectively, as of September 2001 [37].

As the incidence of hematological disorders is rare, if patients on TNF-antagonists develop aplastic anaemia or pancytopenia, these agents should be stopped and patients should be evaluated for evidence of other underlying disease [8].

Leukocytoclastic vasculitis

Mohan et al. [38] described the clinical features of leukocytoclastic vasculitis (LCV) associated with the use of tumor necrosis factor-α (TNF-α) blockers. The Adverse Events Reporting System (AERS) of the US FDA was queried for reports of patients who developed LCV during or after starting etanercept or infliximab from date of approval of each agent through to 6 September 2002.

35 cases of LCV were identified, 20 following etanercept administration and 15 following infliximab administration. 17 of the 35 (48.5%) were biopsy-proven cases and the others had skin lesions that were clinically typical for LCV. 22 of 35 (62.8%) patients had complete or marked improvement of skin lesions upon stopping the TNF-α blocker. Three patients who had received etanercept had continuing lesions despite discontinuation of the drug; one of these patients improved when switched to infliximab. One patient who received infliximab was reported to have continuing lesions despite discontinuation of the drug and treatment with prednisone and antihistamines. 6 patients experienced a positive rechallenge (recurrence of LCV on restarting therapy with a TNF-alpha blocker) and 3 patients a negative rechallenge phenomenon. LCV lesions improved in patients despite continuing use of concomitant medications reportedly associated with LCV.

The authors concluded that therapy with TNF-α blocking agents may be associated with the development of LCV. Skin lesions improved on discontinuation of anti-TNF-α therapy in most patients. Other causes of LCV should be excluded, and evaluation for systemic involvement with appropriate investigations is recommended [38].

Conclusions

Based on the safety data of these agents, Khanna et al. [18] presented the following conclusions and recommendations, which are worthy of careful consideration:

1. Controlled clinical trials of all three TNF-α antagonists have not consistently shown an increased risk of infections compared with RA patients treated with immunosuppressive agents in the pre-anti-TNF-α therapy era, although serious infections have been rarely associated with their use.
2. Reactivation of granulomatous infections is a serious concern with inhibition of TNF-α and appropriate measures should be taken for detection and treatment of latent infection before initiating therapy with all of these agents.
3. Patients should be vaccinated against common encapsulated organisms before the initiation of the TNF-α antagonists.
4. The relationship of TNF-α antagonists to non-Hodgkin's lymphoma is unclear at this time. The biological plausibility of lymphomas associated with immunomodulatory agents, along with the data presented, raises concerns about potential causality. Continued vigilance is warranted until any relationship of these agents to the lymphoproliferative disorders incidence is fully characterized. There is no evidence linking TNF-α antagonists with a higher incidence of solid tumors.
5. TNF-α antagonists should be avoided in patients with pre-existing demyelinating disease.
6. TNF-α antagonists should be avoided in advanced CHF (NYHA Class III–1V) and in patients with NYHA I and II with reduced ejection fraction (<50%). TNF-α antagonists should be used with great caution in NYHA Class I and II with normal ejection fraction.
7. Drug-induced lupus, cutaneous lupus or pancytopenia have rarely been reported with TNF-α antagonists, and patients should be monitored for clinical signs of systemic lupus erythematosus, vasculitis or for pancytopenia.
8. At present there is no evidence implicating TNF-α antagonists with embryotoxicity, teratogenicity or increased pregnancy loss. However, caution, as usual, is warranted.

References

1 Infliximab (Remicade) package insert. Malvern, PA, USA, Centocor Inc., 2005

2 Kavanaugh A, Keenan GF, DeWoody K, Masters P, Hendricks D, Clark J, Harriman G (2001) Long-term follow-up of patients treated with infliximab in all completed clinical trials category [abstract]. *Arthritis Rheum* 46: S173

3 Etanercept (Enbrel) package insert. Thousand Oaks, CA, USA, Amgen Inc. and Wyeth-Ayerst Pharmaceuticals, 2004

4 Adalimumab (Humira) package insert. North Chicago, IL, USA, Abbott Laboratories, 2005

5 Singh G, Ramey DR, Rausch PL, Schettler J (1999) Serious infections in rheumatoid arthritis: relationship to immunosuppressive use [abstract]. *Arthritis Rheum* 42: S242

6 Doran MF, Crowson CS, Pond GR, O'Fallon WM, Gabriel SE (2002) Frequency of infection in patients with rheumatoid arthritis compared with controls: a population-based study. *Arthritis Rheum* 46: 2287–2293

7 FDA Briefing Document. Update on the TNF-alpha blocking agents [online]. Available from URL: http://www.fda.gov/ohrms/dockets/ac/03/briefing/3930b1.htm [Accessed 2003 Sep 1]

8 Furst DE, Breedveld FC, Kalden JR, Smolen JS, Antoni CE, Bijalsma JW, Burmester GR,

Cronstein B, Keystone EC, Kavanaugh A et al (2002) Updated consensus statement on biological agents for the treatment of rheumatoid arthritis and other rheumatic diseases. *Ann Rheum Dis* 61 Suppl. 2: ii2–7
9 Lebwohl M (2002) New developments in the treatment of psoriasis. *Arch Dermatol* 138: 686–688
10 Keane J, Gershon S, Wise RP, Mirabile-Levens E, Kasznica J, Schwieterman WD, Siegel JN, Braun MM (2001) Tuberculosis associated with infliximab, a tumor necrosis factor alpha-neutralizing agent. *N Engl J Med* 345: 1098–1104
11 Bresnihan B, Cunnane G (2003) Infection complications associated with the use of biologic agents. *Rheum Dis Clin North Am* 29: 185–202
12 Gardam MA, Keystone EC, Menzies R, Manners S, Skamene E, Long R, Vinh DC (2003) Anti-tumour necrosis factor agents and tuberculosis risk: mechanisms of action and clinical management. *Lancet Infect Dis* 3: 148–155
13 Keane J, Gershon S (2002) Tuberculosis and treatment with infliximab. *N Engl J Med* 346: 625–626
14 Global tuberculosis control. WHO report: communicable diseases. Geneva: World Health Organisation, 1999
15 Mohan AK, Cote TR, Block JA, Manadan AM, Siegel JN, Braun MM (2004) Tuberculosis following the use of etanercept, a tumor necrosis factor inhibitor. *Clin Infect Dis* 39: 295–299
16 Furst DE, Cush J, Kaufmann S, Siegel J, Kurth R (2002) Preliminary guidelines for diagnosing an treating tuberculosis in patients with rheumatoid arthritis in immunosuppressive trials or being treated with biological agents. *Ann Rheum Dis* 61 Suppl. 2: ii62–63
17 Hamilton CD (2004) Infectious complications of treatment with biologic agents. *Curr Opin Rheumatol* 16: 393–398
18 Khanna D, McMahon M, Furst DE (2004) Safety of tumour necrosis factor-alpha antagonists. *Drug Saf* 27: 307–324
19 Brown SL, Greene MH, Gershon SK, Edwards ET, Braun MM (2002) Tumor necrosis factor antagonist therapy and lymphoma development: twenty-six cases reported to the Food and Drug Administration. *Arthritis Rheum* 46: 3151–3158
20 Wolfe F, Michaud K (2004) Lymphoma in rheumatoid arthritis: the effect of methotrexate and anti-tumor necrosis factor therapy in 18,572 patients. *Arthritis Rheum* 50: 1740–1751
21 Adams AE, Zwicker J, Curiel C, Kadin ME, Falchuk KR, Drews R, Kupper TS (2004) Aggressive cutaneous T-cell lymphomas after TNFalpha blockade. *J Am Acad Dermatol* 51: 660–662
22 http://my.webmd.com/content/article/95/103188.htm. Accessed 21 November 2004
23 http://www.fdaadvisorycommittee.com/FDC/AdvisoryCommittee/Committees/Arthritis±Drugs/030403_TNFsafety/030403_TNFsafetyP.htm. Accessed 21 November 2004
24 Mohan N, Edwards ET, Cupps TR, Oliverio PJ, Sandberg G, Crayton H, Richert JR, Siegel JN (2001) Demyelination occurring during anti-tumor necrosis factor alpha therapy for inflammatory arthritides. *Arthritis Rheum* 44: 2862–2869
25 Kwon HJ, Cote TR, Cuffe MS, Kramer JM, Braun MM (2003) Case reports of heart failure after therapy with a tumor necrosis factor antagonist. *Ann Intern Med* 138: 807–811
26 Debandt M, Vittecoq O, Descamps V, Le Loet X, Meyer O (2003) Anti-TNF-alpha-induced systemic lupus syndrome. *Clin Rheumatol* 22: 56–61
27 Watts RA (2000) Musculoskeletal and systemic reactions to biological therapeutic agents. *Curr Opin Rheumatol* 12: 49–52
28 Maini R, St Clair EW, Breedveld F, Furst D, Kalden J, Weisman M, Smolen J, Emery P, Harriman G, Feldmann M et al (1999) Infliximab (chimeric anti-tumour necrosis factor alpha monoclonal antibody) *versus* placebo in rheumatoid arthritis patients receiving concomitant methotrexate: a randomised phase III trial. ATTRACT Study Group. *Lancet* 354: 1932–1939
29 Rutgeerts P, D'Haens G, Targan S, Vasiliauskas E, Hanauer SB, Present DH, Mayer L, Van Hogezand RA, Braakman T, De Woody KL et al (1999) Efficacy and safety of retreatment with anti-tumor necrosis factor antibody (infliximab) to maintain remission in Crohn's disease. *Gastroenterology* 117: 761–769
30 Shakoor N, Michalska M, Harris CA, Block JA (2002) Drug-induced systemic lupus erythematosus associated with etanercept therapy [letter]. *Lancet* 359: 579–580
31 Stichweh DS, Punaro M, Pascual V (2003) Infliximab-induced double-stranded DNA antibodies in children with rheumatological diseases [abstract]. *Arthritis Rheum* 48: S100
32 Mohan AK, Edwards ET, Cote TR, Siegel JN, Braun MM (2002) Drug-induced systemic lupus erythematosus and TNF-alpha blockers [letter]. *Lancet* 360: 646

33 Bathon JM, Martin RW, Fleischmann RM, Tesser JR, Schiff MH, Keystone EC, Genovese MC, Wasko MC, Moreland LW, Weaver AL (2003) A comparison of etanercept and methotrexate in patients with early rheumatoid arthritis. *N Engl J Med* 343: 1586–1593

34 Zeltser R, Valle L, Tanck C, Holyst MM, Ritchlin C, Gaspari AA (2001) Clinical, histological, and immunophenotypic characteristics of injection site reactions associated with etanercept: a recombinant tumor necrosis factor alpha receptor: Fc fusion protein. *Arch Dermatol* 137: 893–899

35 Wells AF, Kupper H, Fischoff S, Chartash E (2002) Incidence of injection-site reactions association with adalimumab (D2E7) given subcytokine cutaneously for at least 6 months: a retrospective analysis of 4 phase 2/3 clinical trials [abstract]. *Arthritis Rheum* 46: S171

36 Baert F, Noman M, Vermeire S, Van Assche G, D' Haens G, Carbonez A, Rutgeerts P (2003) Influence of immunogenicity on the long-term efficacy of infliximab in Crohn's disease. *N Engl J Med* 348: 601–608

37 ACR Hotline. FDA Advisory Committee Reviews Safety of TNF Inhibitors. Atlanta (GA); American College of Rheumatology, 2001

38 Mohan N, Edwards ET, Cupps TR, Slifman N, Lee JH, Siegel JN, Braun MM (2004) Leukocytoclastic vasculitis associated with tumor necrosis factor-alpha blocking agents. *J Rheumatol* 31: 1955–1958

Index

The MDT-Series Milestones in Drug Therapy

The discovery of drugs is still an unpredictable process. Breakthroughs are often the result of a combination of factors, including serendipidity, rational strategies and a few individuals with novel ideas. *Milestones in Drug Therapy* highlights new therapeutic developments that have provided significant steps forward in the fight against disease. Each book deals with an individual drug or drug class that has altered the approach to therapy. Emphasis is placed on the scientific background to the discoveries and the development of the therapy, with an overview of the current state of knowledge provided by experts in the field, revealing also the personal stories behind these milestone developments. The series is aimed at a broad readership, covering biotechnology, biochemistry, pharmacology and clinical therapy.

Forthcoming titles:

Tamoxifen and Beyond, V.C. Jordan (Author), 2006
Pharmacotherapy of Obesity, J.P.H. Wilding (Editor), 2006
Drugs affecting Growth of Tumours, H.M. Pinedo, C. Smorenburg (Editors), 2006

Published volumes:

Aromatase Inhibitors, B.J.A. Furr (Editor), 2006
Cannabinoids as Therapeutics, R. Mechoulam (Editor), 2005
St. John`s Wort and its Active Principles in Anxiety and Depression, W.E. Müller (Editor), 2005
Drugs for Relapse Prevention of Alcoholism, R. Spanagel, K. Mann (Editors), 2005
COX-2 Inhibitors, M. Pairet, J. Van Ryn (Editors), 2004
Calcium Channel Blockers, T. Godfraind (Author), 2004
Sildenafil, U. Dunzendorfer (Editor), 2004
Hepatitis Prevention and Treatment, J. Colacino, B.A. Heinz (Editors), 2004
Combination Therapy of AIDS, E. De Clercq, A.M. Vandamme (Editors), 2004
Cognitive Enhancing Drugs, J. Buccafusco (Editor), 2004
Fluoroquinolone Antibiotics, A.R. Ronald, D. Low (Editors), 2003
Erythropoietins and Erythropoiesis, G. Molineux, M. Foote, S. Elliott (Editors), 2003

Macrolide Antibiotics, W. Schönfeld, H. Kirst (Editors), 2002
HMG CoA Reduktase Inhibitors, G. Schmitz, M. Torzewski (Editors), 2002
Antidepressants, B.E. Leonard (Editor), 2001
Recombinant Protein Drugs, P. Buckel (Editor), 2001
Glucocorticoids, N. Goulding, R.J. Flower (Editors), 2001z
Modern Immunosuppressives, H.-J. Schuurman (Editor), 2001
ACE Inhibitors, P. D'Orleans-Juste, G. Plante (Editors), 2001
Atypical Antipsychotics, A.R. Cools, B.A. Ellenbroek (Editors), 2000
Methotrexate, B.N. Cronstein, J.R. Bertino (Editors), 2000
Anxiolytics, M. Briley, D. Nutt (Editors), 2000
Proton Pump Inhibitors, L. Olbe (Editor), 1999
Valproate, W. Löscher (Editor), 1999

GPSR Compliance

The European Union's (EU) General Product Safety Regulation (GPSR) is a set of rules that requires consumer products to be safe and our obligations to ensure this.

If you have any concerns about our products, you can contact us on ProductSafety@springernature.com

In case Publisher is established outside the EU, the EU authorized representative is:

Springer Nature Customer Service Center GmbH
Europaplatz 3
69115 Heidelberg, Germany

Batch number: 10584620

Printed by Printforce, the Netherlands